Answers from the Gut

Improving Health and Longevity

SECOND EDITION

John E. Chalmers

Acknowledgments

First, I would like to thank God for giving me the strength to undertake and persevere through all the steps and processes required to bring this project to fruition. Without His blessings, I would not even be here, let alone be able to make this happen.

Over the years, I have interacted with many people with health challenges. My intentions have always been to help however I can. I want to thank those people whose stories I have shared with you. Hopefully their experiences will help the reader as decisions are made going forward.

I talked to several local published authors to gain their insight into what I was getting into. I also had discussions with Lucy tapping her expertise. Their views and comments were very encouraging. One author summarized her opinion by saying "forge ahead". These encouragements mean a lot when a person is moving into unfamiliar territory.

I have had two book editors on this endeavor, Kathy and Marianne. I appreciate their comments and insights which has led to a much better finished product. It's not always easy to take thoughts and ideas and communicate them to the potential audience. Their guidance has been much appreciated.

Maureen at Mo's Art Graphic Design has been wonderful to work with. She has promptly and creatively worked on the book interior charts and graphs as well as the cover design.

My caring and supportive wife, Cheryl, has been with me in this journey of life and the journey to make this book happen. I am thankful every single day for her support and encouragement.

Disclaimer

This book contains the opinion of the author and is not intended to be medical advice. This book will be greatly complemented by discussions with your own medical doctor. A reader should consult their own qualified health care provider for medical advice related to their individual condition.

A reader using or misusing the content of this book does so at reader's own risk and assumes sole responsibility for the outcome they experience. This book is sold and distributed with the understanding that the publisher and author shall have neither liability nor responsibility for any actual or alleged injury that may be caused by application of the contents of this book.

NOTE: In order to maintain the anonymity of individuals and places, some identifying characteristics and details such as names, physical properties, occupations, and places of residence have been changed.

Dedication

To my wife, Cheryl, who has traveled this journey of life and all of its challenges with me for over 50 years.

Life is in some ways like a roller coaster with many ups and downs. For many of those years, the uphill climb from the lows seemed insurmountable, but Cheryl has been supportive and always there, no matter what.

Proverbs 3

Blessed are those who find wisdom, those who gain understanding, for she is more profitable than silver and yields better returns than gold. She is more precious than rubies; nothing you desire can compare with her. Long life is in her right hand; in her left hand are riches and honor. Her ways are pleasant ways, and all her paths are peace. She is a tree of life to those who take hold of her; those who hold her fast will be blessed.

(New International Version (NIV))

Contents

Introduction

The experiences and conclusions that I'm sharing are extremely significant. I have come to the belief that what we eat directly correlates at a higher level than most realize in both our health and longevity. We don't fully realize the consequences of what we eat and the potential opportunity if we change.

This writing will provide the reader with stories and anecdotes of my own experiences on how I arrived at a position of much better health – out of the depths of poor health and a near-death experience. This proved to be a tough journey, but one that has led to some surprisingly and impressive results.

Quite unexpectedly, I discovered solutions to the laundry list of health conditions I endured, from asthma, allergies, arthritis, sinus infections, to psychiatrists when doctors didn't believe me, and finally, to being diagnosed with Crohn's disease. The result is what I believe has general application for others to improve both health and longevity for many people. I not only believe that a sick person like me can become healthier, but that a so-called healthy person can become even healthier.

It is time for people to start taking action to achieve good health and get out of the mode of reacting to health issues after they occur when the damage is already done. While we have impressive technologies in medicines and operations, it's always better not to need them. We want to have the technology around in the case there are unexpected issues, but this shouldn't be the main plan.

Additionally, the big debate in healthcare shouldn't be cost and how to pay for it. What it should be is how best to pursue good health. We as a society should be emphasizing avoiding heart disease, cancer, strokes, and other major diseases. We should be proactive in approaching health through good lifestyle choices including good diet.

I started this quest as an effort born out of desperation to just improve my health and make living more tolerable. I ended up coming to an understanding of how people in general can greatly improve their health and enhance their opportunity for longevity, while at the same time, lowering medical costs. This important information needs to be shared and understood as it is very different from current thinking.

For many years of my life, I thought I was a candidate for the Suffering Hall of Fame, burdened with sickness and disease with no end in sight. Symptom layered upon symptom, illness upon illness, yielding a relentless misery. Every single day felt like punishment for living. With little if any hope for the future, for years it was a challenge just to get through the day.

The bodily damage that occurred through all of this was significant. Operations were performed to remove damaged tissue or to make repairs. Medications were prescribed, but the discouraging long term trends did not stop. In my state of misery, I was on a collision course to future disaster.

But now, life is different. All of the health challenges in the past are gone, and it was a lengthy list. As a senior citizen now, I'm blessed with surprisingly good health compared to my younger bad health years. People found it hard to believe how someone like me who was in such bad shape before, well, how could he improve so much? And some I secretly believe thought maybe I wasn't being honest how ill I was. But I was completely honest, and I was gravely ill.

This brings us to the debate over healthcare, where the most highly publicized issues are twofold: the cost and who is going to pay. The reality for many is that healthcare is too expensive and no longer affordable. My hope in these writings is to show you how the demand or need for medical services can be lowered, leading to lower costs.

My successes and failures have happened within the mainstream of the healthcare system. I didn't venture outside of anything that didn't originate within that establishment. Yet, within the realm of the medical world, there are more options than most people realize by what they eat. The answers are from the gut.

Part One

Chapter 1

Healthcare Costs Over $10,000 per Person

The course we are on as a country concerning healthcare has no good end. Costs have become astronomical. This is a relatively new problem. Advances in medical processes and techniques though bring forth products and services. This caters to what most people believe to be as solutions to their issues.

The Cost to Live

Healthcare costs have risen to the point that they average over $10,000 per person in the United States. That staggering number is presented in a report titled *National Health Expenditure 2016 Highlights* published by the United States Centers for Medicare and Medicaid Services. From that same report, hospital care, physician and clinical services, and prescription drugs account for 62% of spending.

That means that the average cost for a family of four is over $40,000. That's not too far from the total average family income. $10,000 spread out over 330 million people in the United States works out to $3.3 trillion, a huge chunk of our GDP (gross domestic product) or about 18% of our economy and growing at a rate of over 4% per year.

The United States federal government spends about $32 billion on healthcare research and development (R&D).[1] That is a lot of R&D dollars. That spending is geared towards developing innovations in prescription drugs and operations. Additionally, there are many private and not-for-profit organizations also funding and conducting research. This is the money that continually promises to find "cures". We all want cures, right?

The United States has basically entered an era that can be characterized as the *healthcare age*. The *industrial age* that we were in for many years has peaked and is on the decline. Following the industrial age, we went into what was termed the *information age*. Now that we have lots of computers and high technology devices, we've moved towards an era where healthcare is paramount. Our country and its economy now revolve around healthcare.

Cost Per Person

No country on earth spends more per person for healthcare than the United States. It's not even close. While the expenditures on healthcare are high, there are concerns about the resulting outcomes. Given the high levels of R&D and healthcare spending, the U.S. can reasonably expect to have the best care in the world. The question is, do we have the most healthy people who live the longest lives? No, we do not.

The federal government has control of a large portion of the healthcare system through programs such as Medicare. Administrators at Medicare use their clout to fix prices at lower than market rates. By arbitrarily paying for medicines and procedures at a lower level than previously found in the market, our government declares victory at reducing medical costs. Well, not really reducing costs, but reducing the rate of increase.

What is Really Happening

Our federal and state governments in recent years have become more and more involved in healthcare. A major attempt at overhauling a large part of the industry occurred with the passage of the Patient Protection and Affordable Care Act of 2010, also known as Obamacare. Costs though continued to rise and politicians continue to work toward changes.

The healthcare landscape is rapidly changing as a result of federal government actions. In recent years, the trend is for private practice physicians to go the way of dinosaurs in favor of physicians' groups that are often part of hospitals. Hospitals continue to go through mergers, acquisitions, and expansions that further confuses patients needing treatment.

An article in the New York Times titled *When Hospitals Buy Doctors' Offices, and Patient Fees Soar* by Margot Sanger-Katz offers the following explanation:

"Imagine you're a Medicare patient, and you go to your doctor for an ultrasound of your heart one month. Medicare pays your doctor's office $189, and you pay about 20 percent of that bill as a co-payment.

Then, the next month, your doctor's practice has been bought by the local hospital. You go to the same building and get the same test from the same doctor, but suddenly the price has shot up to $453, as has your share of the bill."[2]

The same article further explains:

"Medicare, the government health insurance program for those 65 and over or the disabled, pays one price to independent doctors and another to doctors who work for large health systems — even if they are performing the exact same service in the exact same place."[3]

This clearly shows an example of federal government intervention that is changing the healthcare landscape, and as a result, our economy. These changes have consequences. Doctors no longer report to the patients but report to the physicians group for which they work. Their allegiance now belongs to the management.

Over the decades, doctors have become organized according to their training and experience. A patient's entry point into the system is often with general practitioners (GPs). Now, with insufficient GPs, many see lesser trained nurse practitioners and physician assistants. If the patient has a more involved issue, the GP often refers the person to a specialist. The specialists are organized by the issue's location on the body or diagnosis.

For example, if a person has a skin condition, regardless of the cause, the patient may end up with a dermatologist. A person with a heart condition would be directed to a cardiologist. I look at these specialty areas like silos, each containing a different specialty fully designed to treat these symptoms and conditions.

For example, when my father broke his hip, he was hospitalized for treatment. The specialists studied his case very carefully as he was an elderly man with a heart condition.

Eventually he was cleared for what turned out to be a successful surgery. After the surgery, my father wanted to be on a heart-healthy no-salt-added diet prescribed by his cardiologist during his hospital recovery and rehabilitation. Unfortunately, neither the hospital dietitians or the specialist in charge would go along with it. My Dad's heart surgeon, while sympathetic, would not intervene, so the walls of the medical silos involved in this case were not penetrable.

In fact, the hospital dietician did not admit that a no-salt-added to the food diet existed - only that a low salt diet was available. My Dad knew that he was eating too much salt as the fluid retention in his legs and ankles were increasing. When he returned home and got back on his diet, the fluid went down.

Healthcare Then and Now

Doctors in private practice historically have worked for the patients. They would treat patients and the patients would pay the bills. This is a typical free market system. Patients would balance the costs and results leading to future choices based on past outcomes. With the advent of insurance, the patients or employers mostly paid the insurance company, but still controlled the choice of doctor and providers of medical services. That is changing. Now doctors work for the physicians group as employees. This results as a big change in the doctor-patient relationship.

Unfortunately, the increased intervention by government did not bring with it trends of reduced costs. Costs continue to increase. Additional government involvement so far has not brought with it a lot more healthy people. The big change is that the healthcare industry has more revenue opportunities.

Obamacare initially required everyone to have healthcare insurance or be penalized by the Internal Revenue Service (IRS). This resulted, as intended, in more customers for health insurance. Further aiding in the increase of healthcare insurance coverage for people is federal subsidies for low income folks.

Again, this is more revenue into the system than before.

The politicians kept saying that the healthcare insurance plans available under Obamacare were high quality and affordable, but is it? Here is a true example.

A 64-year-old woman has a history of good health and had no health insurance. She earns too much to get a government subsidy, but both the penalty for not having insurance or the insurance premium would pose a financial hardship, creating a dilemma. She ends up buying an Obamacare healthcare insurance policy and starts paying the monthly premium to avoid the penalty. While in the first year of her newly acquired insurance, she is diagnosed with a melanoma. She is treated for the condition and it's believed that the cancer has not spread.

The cost of the medical procedures is less than the insurance policy deductible of $6,000. That means that all of her medical expenses were out-of-pocket. She works out with the provider a payment plan to pay off the bills as none was covered by the Obamacare insurance. The net result of this cancer survivor's experience is that she paid the full cost of the treatment while additionally bearing the burden of the monthly premiums. This is common.

Most people have insurance for their car which pays for repairs, less the deductible, following a car accident. This type of insurance works as most people in a year don't have accidents resulting in claims. Healthcare is different as almost all people use the system. The price tag has become staggering.

Are There Solutions?

For the long haul, I suggest that the demand for healthcare as we currently know it needs to diminish, while at the same time, the health of the population improves. We need to recognize that when a person is in a position where a cure is needed, it's too late. The focus should be in preventing health problems rather than curing them. Therefore, the outcome of improving health and reducing the need for the present healthcare system should result in a longer, higher quality life.

Politicians also talk about having solutions or propose solutions to high and rising healthcare costs to society. With the present paradigms, there realistically is no solution going down the path we're going. Something(s) must change. Innovation or doing something vastly different is required. Right now, people are faced with years of the same.

The medical establishment would transform if a lot of people didn't need it. The whole system would change and those changes would be dramatic. Costs would go down. Supply would better match demand. The advantage in the system would shift toward the consumer. Healthier people would inherently need fewer prescription drugs and operations. Money spent for health-related issues could be spent in other, more desirable ways.

When demand is high and exceeds supply, prices for medical care will likely go up. Increases of government regulations and prices will likely go up. The trend has been for medical costs to rise at a rate faster than inflation with no end in sight. Big problem!

The stakeholders in our healthcare system include the providers, the payers, and the patients. The least organized of the stakeholders is patients themselves. We live in a society that offers us the opportunity to take more responsibility for our health in order to become less dependent on others. That I think is the best choice for each of us.

I have reversed the health trend of my life, sick in the past and healthier now. The good news though is what happened to me can happen to many.

Chapter 2

Resetting the Goal

I propose changing our health goal from finding a cure to becoming so healthy that the body's risk for getting diseases and illnesses is significantly reduced. Going along with improved health is extended lifespans. Today, we've been counting on the medical system to be a primary source of increasing the length of our lives. That needs to change. If we had a clear direction, many of us would make greater efforts to do things that make a difference.

Therefore, the only way left to reduce healthcare costs is to reduce the need for it by finding ways to be healthier. Healthy people need minimal healthcare expenditures.

What is needed is for one's own body to rise to the occasion to fend off illness and disease with a resulting minimal need for medical interventions. So, the health goals (not healthcare goals) become:

1. Be so healthy that medications and operations are not needed for health-related conditions through most of a lifetime.
2. Be so healthy that life expectancy is extended. The extended life brings with it a high-level quality of life requiring little or no help from doctors.
3. Use medical tests (such as blood tests) primarily to verify good health.

Today, healthcare is generally a reactive system. The typical steps are simply to get treatment after one gets sick. When illness shows up, off to the doctor we go. The doctors go through their steps, give a diagnosis, and prescribe the treatment, often a prescription. If the diagnosis is not arrived at through a physical examination, then tests are often ordered to help in the data-gathering to zero in on the diagnosis.

The new steps for the future, to start with, is to be healthy but go in to see the doctor once every year or two for a review of a few tests taken in advance of the visit. The physician reviews the results and confirms there are no unexpected findings, and the patient is good to go for another couple of years.

I have had multiple operations over the years and have taken many prescription medications. Pretty costly, but it was mostly covered by insurance. It's good news that insurance paid for most of it, right? But what I really wanted was to be healthy. Being sick really interferes with life!

Medications and Surgery

Wouldn't we really want to be so healthy that we don't need prescriptions or operations? Wouldn't it be better to not use the insurance we have? Wouldn't it be great to be so healthy and feel so good that a pharmacy in the medicine cabinet is not needed? And not sliced and diced up by highly skilled and trained surgeons?

That thought goes upstream against experience. Most believe that as we get older, medical needs increase. More operations and medications are needed for older people compared to younger ones. It would be great if the really healthy portion of life could be extended to delay the onset of health problems until much later in life.

I have been a sick person, like many others, and have a history of taking medications and surgeries to keep going. Keep me going they did, but certainly not successful in transforming me into a healthy person. The "system" is not geared to making me so healthy that I don't need drugs and surgeries. In fact, there seems to be a greater number of people than ever that are on maintenance doses of medications.

In order to become healthy, the root cause of illness must be found and effectively dealt with. In the absence of finding the root cause, we often treat just the symptoms. There are many diseases that the medical system still doesn't understand regarding the causes and best treatments in dealing with the symptoms.

As I've gotten older, I've given more and more thought to the prospects of wanting to live to a much older age. Most people would like to live a high quality of life for a very long time - me included. The dilemma I faced is I've been sick all of my life with various maladies, with one considered to be an incurable, debilitating disease. You would think that I'd be on many prescriptions given my history, but I arrived at age 70 prescription free. The doctors - I have two of them - could find no reason to prescribe anything. I haven't used over-the-counter medications for years either. My goal years ago was just to get better, healthier someday, some way, somehow. What is "totally healthy"? To me, it was being so healthy to not need any assistance from doctors. A person could be very active and do things they wanted to do. No prescription medications and no operations needed. Good high-quality years of longevity.

Given the progress that has been made in medical technology over the last few hundred years, you would think we could expect developments in terms of raising the level of health for people. Innovation is the word. We're innovating better operations and medicines, but are we innovating better health? Let's stop and think through this for a moment.

There has been a lot of advances in surgeries. Many years ago, there were high mortality rates for many surgeries as technologies were crude by today's standards. The high mortality rates for surgery led to advances and levels of continuous improvements with doctors and scientists striving for improved results. As these incremental improvements in technology immerged, mortality rates declined.

Let's take the case of blocked arteries to the heart. Suppose a person is diagnosed with this and bypass surgery is recommended. Surgery is undertaken and the patient recovers. The surgical procedure and the result are closely tied together as the action and result are linked. Years ago, this surgery was not possible. If bypass surgery was tried a hundred years ago, the patient would surely die as the technology for a successful result did not yet exist. It has evolved to the point now that it's commonly done and the risks are pretty low. This is an example of lifespans being extended through medical science.

Operations, while certainly not cures, are becoming more and more effective in dealing with damage to the body. In 1882, Dr. William Halsted performed the first successful surgery to remove gallstones on his own mother.[4] Previously, the patient's most likely prognosis was death. Today, gallbladder surgery is routine with recovery times short and success rates very high. Progress in surgeries over the last 130 years is very impressive, and one great benefit is immediate results.

Surgery and associated techniques are wonderful for cases resulting from injuries. Suffer an injury and the medical community has a lot to offer. Then there are operations for cases like the blocked artery in the heart mentioned previously. What if the heart disease doesn't occur though? The need for the associated operations would be eliminated, or at least minimized.

Unlike surgeries, causes for many diseases are disconnected from the health result. Take for example an alcoholic where excessive drinking increases the likelihood of liver disease. People can abuse their body for years and later serious problems can emerge. But, for many years, the alcoholic seems to be "getting away" with the behavior because the damage is gradual.

Cures vs. Prevention

The National Foundation for Infantile Paralysis (NFIP) at one time was raising huge amounts of money to find the "cure" for polio. To me, a cure is when one has the disease or disorder and a means (the cure) is found to restore health. As far as I know, once polio is contracted, there remains no cure. The vaccines that were developed are given to healthy people in the hope that the result would be immunity to contracting the disease. Today, virtually no one contracts polio.

This is a pretty important concept. There are lots of diseases that once contracted cannot be cured. That has led to the idea of having many vaccinations to prevent the disease from occurring.

What if people were to be so healthy that their bodies effectively dealt with diseases without medicines (including vaccinations)? People would develop natural immunities without medicine intervening. An example of a great breakthrough in medicine has been the development of antibiotics. President Calvin Coolidge's son incurred a blister on his foot that became infected. Despite receiving all the treatment that medical science could offer at the time, Calvin junior passed away at the age of 16.[5] The best doctors in the world in the 1920's couldn't help young Coolidge for what today is a minor condition when treated with antibiotics.

As great as antibiotics are, there is a downside. Antibiotics have been so successful that we constantly hear stories of how they're over prescribed. This has resulted in some cases of lowering its effectiveness of certain antibiotics for some disorders.

I have taken many medications in my life and I can assure you that none have produced a cure for me. In fact, most have had the effectiveness of a spoonful of water. In some cases, I dealt with unpleasant side effects. Far too often it proved to be a waste of time. I took them anyway because there was no alternative or nowhere else to turn.

Are We Living Longer?

An article by Mike Strobes titled, *No Clear Cause of Drop in US Life Expectancy* tells us the reason people live longer has historically been due to "medical advances, public health campaigns, and better nutrition and education."[6]

So, with all the advances in surgery and medicine, life expectancy should continue to go up, right? It's unfortunate, but in spite of all these advances, lifespans are no longer increasing.

The following table explains in more detail.

YEAR	LIFE EXPECTANCY AT BIRTH (YEARS)	INFANT MORTALITY % (0 TO 1 YEAR)
1901	49.2	12.4
1939-41	63.6	4.7
1959-61	69.7	1.0
1989-91	75.4	0.9
2012	78.8	0.6
2013	78.8	0.6
2014	78.9	0.6
2015	78.8	0.6
2016	78.7	0.6

Table 2.1. Data from United States Life Tables as published by the National Center for Health Statistics.

In understanding this table, it's important to know that "life expectancy at birth" refers to the expected average age at death for people born in the Year column shown in the table.

Notice how life expectancy at birth steadily climbed for over 100 years. Notice the correlation to infant mortality (death within the first year of birth) that shows a dramatic decline. It's safe to say that as infant mortality went down, the age of life expectancy at birth went up.

But in recent years, the life expectancy at birth seems to have hit a plateau, with life expectancy averaging in at 78.8 years during that period.[7]

Societal changes have contributed to longer life spans. There's been a large decrease in the use of tobacco. Asbestos has been virtually eliminated. The development of antibiotics and improved surgeries definitely contribute to longer life spans. Often overlooked contributors to increased lifespans are improved water quality, personal hygiene, and sewage handling. These coupled with some other factors along with major decreases in infant mortality account for much of the improvement.

My late grandmother told me once that pregnant moms in the early 1900's stayed in the hospital for three weeks before returning home with their babies! This most likely happened due to the high infant mortality rate of that era. Today, moms are in and out of the hospital often in one day. Long hospital stays apparently were not a difference maker; rather, cleanliness made a difference - in safer drinking water, personal hygiene, and advancements in the sterilization of hospital equipment.

To be fair in assessing the leveling out of life expectancy at birth in recent years, some areas that could be contributing to this is the dramatic increase in overweight or obese children and adults. Our country is also knee deep into a drug use epidemic.

In the next chapter, some background and an approach will be laid out to provide an understanding and roadmap towards exceptional health and well-being while reducing healthcare expenses and increasing longevity.

Chapter 3

Emphasize Prevention for Healthcare

We often think of a healthcare system as the various resources used to return people with health issues toward good health. Doctors, hospitals, and health-related equipment have all been developed towards that end. The healthcare system of which we have been so proud of is one which emphasizes using resources such as medical doctors and medicines.

Tremendous resources are in place, but what is being achieved? Develop a better medicine, a better operation, or a better test is what seems to be the main thrust of advancing healthcare for people. In an ideal world, what should we really be trying to achieve? It would seem like an unbelievable objective for people to live without the need for medical intervention and yet live longer than expected today. Wouldn't it be great if people lived a long time and needed no medical interventions, or at least until years later in life? Some do, but in the United States, it's not many. It's hard to imagine a world where people are so healthy that they don't need prescriptions or other treatments except for injuries.

With healthcare costs so high in the United States, is there a way to reduce these costs while at the same time, have people healthier than ever and satisfied that their needs are being met?

The high level of controversy on this subject makes it seem like there is no clear path to lower costs and greater accessibility. Yet, in other industries, costs go down while the quality of goods and services rise.

Comparing Healthcare to Other Industries

People who are in the business of manufacturing - the products we use every day, continuously look for ways to produce high quality items at low costs with few issues. Over the years, the quality and reliability of products we buy has risen while costs have gone down.

For example, years ago, televisions needed repairs fairly often. There was a vast network of television repairmen throughout the country who often made house calls to fix them. All of the drug stores had tube testers for those adventuresome enough to try to replace the individual television tubes when they failed. Gone are the tubes and tube testers, replaced with high tech components and circuitry on printed circuit boards. Today, televisions provide a much better picture quality and are much more reliable. Television repair shops still exist but are few and far between. The landscape in the world of television has changed and quality through innovation has gone up while prices have gone down.

It would be great for people to have a small need for the healthcare system and live long quality lives just as our television sets do today compared to the past. My grandfather at 25 years old was told by his family doctor that he had approximately six months to live due to the discovery of a heart murmur. For the rest of his life, the only reason he went to a medical doctor was to satisfy the requirement for an annual physical required by his employer. He lived to the age of 93 years - 68 years without prescriptions and other medical interventions that are so common today. I think that he might have lived longer with medical help in his last few years, but his longevity was impressive.

The United States healthcare system is one with rising costs with rising use. When a person suffers an injury, the technology our medical community can offer is wonderful compared to years past. This area has advanced with the result being saved lives and quality of life improvements.

Inspection Costs

Within this world, many procedures really amount to inspections and tests. People are checked for blood pressure and heartbeat rate. X-rays and blood tests are common. New medical tests (inspections) are developed frequently. When a person goes in for a checkup, it's an inspection to see if any conditions can be detected. People are generally sold on the idea of a checkup as a way to detect a condition early with the belief that early detection will offer a better prognosis.

Inspection costs in the product manufacturing world are costs associated with product measurement and evaluation, similar to what is done in the healthcare arena. Inspections made as a part of the production process could be minimal in expense or could be major dollars in relation to the cost of producing a product. An example of an inspection in manufacturing might be measuring the size of a product to make sure it conforms to customer specifications or requirements.

Like the product manufacturing case, when a person is given a medical test (inspection), there are generally two outcomes: the person fails the test or passes. Passing a test could have two outcomes though. It can indicate no issues, or it might point to the need to do additional tests if symptoms still exist. Failing the test indicates the person has a problem or condition and further intervention may be needed. The right kind of test (inspection) becomes important here.

Failure Costs

In the healthcare realm, medical bills for treatment of illness, disease, and/or injury are examples of what manufacturing people call failure costs. For purposes of this discussion, once a person has a disease or illness, a failure (to be healthy) has occurred. Once the diagnosis is made, the reaction to failure is often a medication, operation, or other treatment. The treatment resulting from the diagnosis is truly failure costs. It should always be preferred to be healthy and not need medical treatment. Now let's make the analogy with producing something in the manufacturing environment.

When defective units are made, rework and scrap are examples of failures. An example of a failure cost in a production environment is a drip or run occurring when a part has been painted. The drip or run in the paint not acceptable to the customer could require sanding and repainting to correct. This is an example of "not right the first time", and an extra cost (due to a failure) is incurred to bring the product to a level that is acceptable for sale.

Back to healthcare, if a person is diagnosed with a problem artery that doctors say require surgery, the failure is the problem artery. The failure costs would be associated with the operation and/or medication required to deal with it. If the artery never had the issue, the medical intervention would not be needed and no failure costs would occur. This is the ideal case where good health and low healthcare costs occur simultaneously.

Failure costs and inspection costs often increase together. Tests and evaluations (inspection costs) are needed for diagnosis and monitoring of conditions as people are being treated (failure costs).

Quality Assurance

Now let's introduce the idea of true prevention. If a person has a heart attack, inspection and failure costs will be incurred. If the heart attack happened, it can no longer be prevented. Prevention as defined here are the activities to keep failures from happening. The problems or failures have yet to happen which provides an opportunity to prevent their occurrence.

In the manufacturing environment, prevention techniques have been in place for many years. There are costs associated with prevention activities, but the payoffs have historically been huge, relatively speaking, by reducing inspection and failure costs. The old adage that applies here is "an ounce of prevention is worth a pound of cure".

In manufacturing, prevention may take the form of quality planning. Quality plans can contain the steps and precautions used to produce quality production while minimizing potential problems. The emphasis here is on potential problems...problems that have never happened but might occur in the future. This is often done starting with evaluations at the product design stage and at all stages of the process to successfully deliver a product. It meets or exceeds a customer's expectations with minor issues along the way. Prevention is clearly thinking through matters ahead of time.

Making the analogy to people is more challenging. Most of what we call today as prevention is not prevention. A person who gets an annual check-up is really getting an inspection. While this check-up is often called a preventive measure, it is really a way to detect a health issue (failure) or the absence of a health issue at an early stage.

What systems are in place that help people live long, healthy, quality lives while healthcare interventions (inspections failure costs) are minimized?

Education is one way. What constitutes a healthy lifestyle could be prevention via knowledge. Of course, there would need to be action associated with the education for it to be effective.

Is There a Science to Staying Healthy?

Scientists have developed some insights into actions that people can take to be healthy. The forces of the marketplace probably make the message muddled and unclear. Messages are bombarded upon us daily presenting alternatives for good health. We constantly hear about exercise and exercise devices as well as a multitude of diet programs. Sorting through the possibilities is pretty much impossible.

Additionally, there is more than one approach to the same issue coming from the scientific community. An example is the placement of babies in their cribs while sleeping to avoid sudden infant death syndrome (SIDS). Over the years, those recommendations have changed.

By the definitions above though, most if not all of our healthcare costs are in the inspection and failure categories. In the area of prevention, there's very little available to people outside of the obvious. For example, overexposure to the sun can result in sunburn, or even worse, skin cancer. This type of cancer known as melanoma can be prevented by avoiding prolonged sun exposure.

We often hear that exercise can be good for us, however, it's unclear what the optimal level of exercise is for good health. We're told that the air we breathe can be a problem. Over the years, the air quality has steadily improved in the U.S. from pollution.

To look at an example of the not-so-obvious, the U. S. government at one time had a Food Pyramid, a recommended listing of foods for a so-called healthy diet. It has been modified over time and even renamed as MyPlate. Regardless of the name, the U.S. Department of Agriculture has been under some criticism for its recommendations. Yes, we still don't have a universal agreement of foods to eat for good health!

Prevention when applied to the health of people is a real opportunity. In the manufacturing world, when prevention activities are increased, it's very common for costs to go down as less is spent towards inspections and failures. My experience is that the same results could happen for the healthcare of people. Shifting the healthcare emphasis to prevention could result in healthier people who need fewer inspections (tests and evaluations) or failures (health issues).

A huge paradigm shift would be required to move towards prevention. This change has already occurred in many manufacturing companies. Quality planning and other prevention tools are now commonplace. In healthcare, the future might include a quality of life plan leading to lower costs much like what has happened in manufacturing. Could preventative measures possibly come from the gut?

The feasibility of actually laying out a game plan for good health and longevity is not rare. I looked around for an example which demonstrates this concept and found one fairly easily. Although not the approach I would put at the top of my list, it's an approach well documented that shows great results.

The dietary/lifestyle approach I discovered comes from the Seventh-Day Adventist Church, a Christian Protestant denomination well known for its Sabbath day falling on Saturdays (which they view is the 7th day of the week). The church was established in 1863 in Battle Creek, Michigan. One of the church's founders was Ellen G. White, whose influence through her prolific writings remains to this day. Also heavily involved early in the church was John Harvey Kellogg, M.D., who along with his brother, Will, invented corn flakes. Dr. Kellogg founded the business now known as the Kellogg Company, headquartered in Battle Creek. Kellogg shared the Seventh Day

Adventist belief in a vegetarian diet, abstaining from alcohol and tobacco, and endorsing regular exercise.

The lifestyle espoused by the Seventh-Day Adventists seems to have originated with Ellen G. White, who told of visions she experienced, and ultimately led some people to believe that she was a messenger of God. These visions included the subject of health and well-being.

A very detailed book documenting data and studies comparing Adventist populations with non-Adventist populations is the book, *Diet, Life Expectancy, and Chronic Disease: Studies of Seventh-Day Adventists and Other Vegetarians* by Gary E. Fraser. Fraser presented many study results that indicated improved longevity for the Adventist lifestyle.

His results indicated that Adventist men who live to age 30 years live 7.28 years longer, while women live 4.42 years longer.[8] In another study, Fraser reported that men lived 9.5 years longer while women lived 6.1 years longer.[9] For the Adventist population, in addition to increased longevity, the onset of serious illnesses still occurred but showed up later in life.[10]

Here we have a documented example of people living longer through lifestyle choices. Avoiding smoking and drinking along with getting some exercise are important choices to good health for everyone.

With that in mind, the remainder of this book discusses the diet (nourishment) portion of the formula to longevity and good health.

Part Two

Chapter 4

My Childhood and Early Adult Years

While growing up, I constantly used the healthcare system. Being sickly from childhood brought with it many challenges and frustrations. Bronchial asthma, hay fever, and pneumonia dominated throughout my adolescent years. Being chronically sick is a more accurate way to describe it.

One doctor told my mother that he felt I would get healthier if I was able to just get through childhood. With this kind of personal history, there was always the dream of being healthy and not needing to go to doctors or taking medicine.

I was a sickly skinny kid. Many trips were made to the doctor with school days missed. I was characterized as a bronchial asthmatic with spells of coughing, wheezing, and difficulty breathing. These symptoms sometimes came upon me often for no apparent reason, or during moderate or strenuous physical activity. My breathing became very labored if I was around animals, so I avoided them whenever possible. Dust was a big problem.

I also had significant hay fever (allergic rhinitis) symptoms. My hay fever symptoms would start in the spring and last until the hard frosts in the fall. While other kids my age enjoyed the summer months away from school, I stayed indoors suffering from severe nasal congestion, runny nose, and watery eyes. The treatment for hay fever didn't amount to much. Antihistamines helped a bit, but I felt tired and drained all the time from the side effects.

In three separate years following my routine hay fever symptoms, I contracted pneumonia that I suspect was caused by my weakened condition. One of those years I spent a week in the hospital. But once my sick season passed, I did pretty well if I avoided dust and animals.

When I joined the Army, I filled out forms indicating my health history. The Army took me because in those days, the main requirement to get in was just being alive and breathing.

My cousin, who was totally blind in one eye, was accepted as well. He made it through basic training until the rifle range activities started when luckily for his fellow service members he didn't pass and was discharged out!

I went into basic training and everything seemed to be going fairly well until we started to run distances. Early in that process, I had a wheezing spell and was taken to a base doctor. He told me on the spot that I had two choices: remain in the Army but not be allowed to participate in any physical training or activity, or begin the process to be discharged. I ended up being honorably discharged and returned home. I couldn't make it through basic training.

Little did I know as I entered adulthood that more health challenges were coming.

Several years later, more symptoms started to set in. First came the diarrhea which gradually intensified. In addition, abdominal pain and chills set in. The level of distress varied somewhat but was always there, every single day. Sometimes it would feel tolerable and sometimes I was doubled over in pain.

I had no days free of symptoms. It was akin to being tortured.

I went to the family doctor. After listening about my symptoms, he told me that I had a condition due to nerves. He prescribed no medications and he sent me on my way. He didn't seem sympathetic to my problems. I was stunned at getting no help from this doctor! I didn't know what to do next.

My condition gradually went from bad to worse. I was deteriorating, losing weight. I went back to the doctor again. I was more insistent this time and he prescribed some pills. I could hardly wait to get to the pharmacy to get the prescription filled. Unfortunately, the pills had no impact. This was demoralizing.

As the year progressed, it was getting harder and harder for me to get through a day. I would go to work using all the mental and physical strength I could muster. After the work day, I would get home drained of energy and would just collapse. I often wondered why I had to suffer so much. Why me?!

Ordinary tasks became difficult. I was trying to put up a front to the world that I was okay when really I was not. I felt trapped. I concentrated my energy and drew from within to try to get through a day. There were no moments to savor the flowers, the birds, and the sky. There were no moments of tranquility. I found that I had to keep busy and the distress lessened a little bit or maybe it was just more tolerable. Any idle time turned into a virtual collapse for me.

Getting no help from my doctor, I decided to try an exercise program at my wife's suggestion. I was losing weight and there was the thought that it might help me add some pounds. At the time, as bad as I felt, I wasn't very excited about trying this but decided to give it a chance. To be honest, I didn't know how I would have the energy to do it.

I was set up with an exercise program at a fitness center and was encouraged to hear that some people had gained weight. I tried to look at this endeavor as a very positive step.

I went to the fitness center 3 days a week. I felt like the classic 90-pound weakling and didn't weigh much more among the muscular instructors and body building patrons. My muscles started to feel pretty good. I was not gaining weight though nor were my symptoms improving.

After a few months on the exercise program, it was time for progress measurements. While I was definitely getting stronger in terms of the weights I could lift, no body weight gain was measured. I remained very ill.

One of the instructors tried to sell me some weight gain food supplements that he was selling on a commission basis. In the process of trying to sell me the supplements, he made some rough comments about my physique which I took pretty hard. I just felt like beating my head against the wall in frustration.

If fitness training by itself had been the answer, I think I would have found it there, but that was not the case. Several years into the suffering, I relocated to another city for a job with a different company. One of my motives was access to the additional medical resources the new larger city had to offer.

I continued to struggle to get through a day. The job allowed me some flexibility in that I was free to move about the offices and the manufacturing facility. Except for my

25

underweight condition, it's unlikely anyone noticed how much I was struggling.

By this time, I would've been unable to perform many occupations in the workplace. I couldn't have been a factory worker, a construction worker, or many other labor jobs. I would've been disabled. I was borderline in a work environment that was well suited to my health condition, but I was scared. My family was counting on me. Without my job and its income, I don't know what would have happened to us.

Very quickly, an appointment was made with a new family doctor in the new city. He ran me through a battery of tests. Unfortunately, all of the tests came in negative. Nothing was found to be wrong with me.

Upper GI's (gastrointestinal), Lower GI's, and blood tests were among the tests that revealed no clues. I was miserable every single moment of every single day with health issues. How could there not be a medical reason!

Since none of the tests led to a diagnosis other than "normal", this led me to believe that the diagnosis of "nerves' or "stress-related" might be correct although I still found it hard to believe. The doctor suggested that I make an appointment at a mental health center, which I did.

I met with a psychologist for months. Again, no progress. I was sick and getting sicker. She recognized that she wasn't helping me and suggested that biofeedback training be tried. She set me up with another psychologist who specialized in it.

I knew very little about biofeedback training. A friend who'd contracted multiple sclerosis bought a biofeedback device shortly after learning he had this serious disease in the hopes it would help him. The device didn't work for him, but I was still hopeful since my illness was different.

The Breakthrough

The new psychologist was very personable and good to talk to. He asked questions to build an understanding of my struggles and condition. I was introduced over several sessions to biofeedback machines. I was connected to the machine with the goal being for me to change the response of a bodily activity through my thought process. I was not good at this.

After a while he introduced me to these adhesive-backed round black stickers that were slightly less than a quarter inch in diameter. These little round black stickers or "dots" would change color with body temperature changes. They operated much like the mood rings which were a fad in the 1970s that would also change color with changes in body temperature.

The normal color for the dots was black at room and normal body temperature. I was instructed to put one of the dots on the back of my hand and to try, using my mind, to cause it to change color. I tried very hard but had no success.

Next it was suggested that I keep one dot on my hand at all times to see what would happen. That turned out in my view to be a stroke of genius. About half an hour before my next meal, that little dot seemed to all by itself change colors. That turned out to be the pattern. Shortly before all meals, the little dot would change color.

I was never able through my thought process to change the color. Something about the anticipation of eating a meal though had a dramatic effect.

I didn't understand what was happening, but I did start to feel a little better. A slight weight gain and a small reduction in symptoms occurred without me doing anything different. After this small measure of progress, the psychologist discontinued the office visits. I was not very happy about this as I still had all my symptoms although a little bit reduced. I suppose that I had gotten all biofeedback training had to offer, but physically, I was still in trouble.

Over the next year, my health again gradually started going the wrong way. Symptoms became more intense and my body weight continued to drop. The magic from the little black dots diminished until there was no effect at all.

Small issues became big issues. For example, the brand of deodorant that I'd been using was discontinued by the manufacturer. Not giving it a second thought, I went to the store and just bought a different kind. The next day, I applied it which irritated my skin. I bought another brand and got the same result. I needed a new approach.

The third time I went to the store, I looked for ones that had the fewest ingredients. This took a lot of time, but the one I chose didn't cause skin irritation.

My sensitivities to my environment were greater than I realized. Little did I know that I was entering the year of The Crash.

Chapter 5

The Crash

In late March and early April of the year of my big health crash, I started to have stiffness and pain in my neck. Normal motions of my head were uncomfortable and hurt. My left and right turning motions were impaired. It seemed to get a little worse each day but was still tolerable. Then one morning when I woke up, I couldn't get up out of bed. Any movement at all was horrible.

With my wife's assistance, I was eventually able to get out of bed and into a chair. It took a long time to make the transition to the chair, and finally there, I could do nothing. Any movement caused such severe pain that I didn't think I could make it through the day.

Into the hospital I went. It was shortly before Easter and there I was, flat on my back in the hospital. Our family doctor recommended a doctor of internal medicine.

The new doctor came by and reviewed my health history information. In addition to the current neck issue, I wasn't in very good shape. Other routine unexplained symptoms caused a lot of discomfort and difficulty. We're going on nine years of this at this point. I felt overwhelmed.

I went through all kinds of tests. I passed them all. The x-rays of my neck were not conclusive.

The diagnosis eventually arrived. I was told it was likely ankylosing spondylitis (AS), an inflammation of the vertebrae in the back and neck, which can lead to permanent damage, such as fusion of the spine. He prescribed a non-steroidal anti-inflammatory drug (NSAID) called Indocin. At the time, I looked upon this as a high-powered aspirin. The potential side effects of this were pretty scary, but the pills did offer some relief.

Years later, I met a person who had a more significant version of AS than I had. Wayne had worked as an accountant before becoming disabled. The AS resulted in most of his spine being totally stiff. The pain phase had passed so that was not a problem. However, to turn to look to the left, Wayne had to turn his whole body to the left; the same for looking to the right. He was able to sit and stand on his own with a cane, go down a stairway but in a backwards position, but couldn't drive due to the limitations of not being able to move his head.

My neck still hurt some, but unlike Wayne, I was now able to function. The doctor still kept me in the hospital over Easter weekend, even though I wanted to go home.

To treat the rest of my undiagnosed symptoms, my new doctor recommended that I see a psychiatrist. Two psychologists before, now a psychiatrist that I didn't believe was going to help with chills, weight loss, and to say it nicely, a poorly functioning digestive system. I was desperate with no real alternatives, so I gave it a try, and was able to go back to work. I was marginally able to work in my white-collar profession. I couldn't drive at times but could arrange rides when needed. For most lines of work, I would've been considered unable to work and disabled. I needed help to get better soon.

I started to see the psychiatrist on a regular basis. He would ask a lot of questions. We would have discussions over the next several months but there was no progress. In fact, my condition continued to decline. I remember my weight dropping steadily from 130 lbs. to the 120's and on down to 115 lbs. Did I mention that I'm 6 feet tall? During this time, all symptoms other than my neck being controlled by the medications continued to worsen.

In later years, my co-workers told me they thought I was dying. I looked like a walking skeleton. It took all my strength to work.

Early in August, the psychiatrist put me on some medication. I didn't really understand its function but was eager for any relief. My weight was slipping more and I ventured down to 110 lbs. The medication had an immediate impact though. The chills stopped.

My digestive system seemed to function better as some of the symptoms improved. I felt pretty good for a couple of days, better than I had felt for a long time. During my next visit to the psychiatrist, I reported the significant relief of symptoms. It was the first time in a little over nine years that I was feeling better. I didn't realize at the time that I was in the eye of a coming storm.

The Final Crash

Within a week of starting the medication, my symptoms came back with a vengeance. The neck pain remained tolerable but all of my other symptoms had never been so bad. My whole body was in turmoil. I was able to get to work but once there, was useless. I didn't know what was happening or what to expect. I was in serious trouble and knew it.

With my body in chaos, I started having severe abdominal pains on my left side - one intolerable pain followed by another minutes later. These pains doubled me over. Doctors told me my symptoms were psychological. I called my psychiatrist.

His answering service notified him of my call and he returned it. How rude and inconsiderate he was and couldn't understand why I called him! He told me to call my doctor. I could have screamed.

I was put back in the hospital. My family doctor sent a surgeon to visit me. After reviewing my history, he suggested that it was possible I had Crohn's disease. I had no clue what that was. This was the first time a doctor suggested that I had a bona fide medical disorder.

The surgeon's recommendation was to do some exploratory surgery. While lying in the hospital, my abdominal pain had subsided. I didn't take this surgeon's advice and they released me from the hospital. This was a big mistake.

Over the next couple of days, I started to put on a little weight. Then I started not sleeping well. It worsened each night. Then one night I was unable to sleep at all and was up all night. I prayed for the ability to sleep a little and went to work the next day. I couldn't maintain my balance. I called my family doctor, explained what was happening, and he told me to go straight to an x-ray lab.

The doctor had given the staff a heads up about me and I got in right away. They quickly had results and the place started to buzz. Phone calls were being made. I couldn't make out what was being said.

A staff member came out and told me that I had a problem and should go straight to the hospital where the surgeon would meet me in the emergency room. The hospital was just a few minutes away.

The surgeon was there to meet me. He looked at the x-ray results and told me that my condition was dangerous. He said my intestine was totally blocked. There could be gangrene. There was a potential to lose the entire colon. My head spun. I was admitted.

I was in such bad shape that he couldn't operate immediately. He prescribed some enemas for a few days to try and open the blockage and improve my health. The enemas did help the suffering but did nothing for the blockage.

I was able to sleep and they hooked me up to IVs and oxygen. I prayed a lot in that hospital bed. I knew I was in crisis. I was afraid. Then my thought process changed. After realizing that I was praying for myself, I prayed that I would commit to doing good things and find ways to help other people if I made it through. An immediate peace came over me. I couldn't control the future. My life was in God's hands.

My fears subsided. I was ready for the surgery.

The doctor came in the second day and told me the surgery would happen the next day no matter what. He could wait no longer.

The efforts to improve my condition had failed. While being wheeled into the operating room, the beehive of activity as the doctors and nurses busily prepared sunk in. The lights were bright and frightening. The anesthesiologist came over and talked to me, telling me that soon he would ask me to count from 100 backwards. I made it to 98.

When I woke up, it seemed like only a few minutes later. I had a tube down my nose into my stomach to keep it drained and could only suck on ice. Some device or machine seemed to be attached to me from all angles. Three feet of large intestines and one foot of small intestine were removed until healthy tissue was found. I could get up to walk the next day. I'll tell you, walking was not what I felt like doing! To manage the pain from the surgery, I was given shots in the hip that felt almost as bad.

I held off on the next one as long as I could, but each walk did help the pain with the nurses assisting me.

As I laid in my hospital room hoping that I was recovering, I started thinking about a local news anchor who had recently died. There were some sketchy reports that she had some kind of intestinal infection. The doctors kept removing bowel sections through operations. They failed to save her though, a once vibrant, attractive woman who had the potential to work for a one of the major networks. Could that be me too?

I had no idea what caused my problems. Now I had multiple doctors checking on me daily - my family doctor, the internalist, the psychiatrist or his assistant, and the surgeon. The surgeon came twice a day. He was very particular with staff that everything had to be just right for me, and I appreciated his caring attitude.

The psychiatrist also came around almost daily. One day his assistant came in alone. Neither of them ever said much – just looked at my chart, said a few words and left. Then I found out why after getting a big bill for services while I was recuperating. Needless to say, I never had anything to do with him again. He was nothing short of a crook taking advantage of me.

My Recovery

As I laid in the hospital, I felt stronger each day in spite of my weight being around 100 pounds. I started to realize that I was going to make it. I was going to survive. My bowel function did not start on its own, so the surgeon ordered medication to get it going. It worked. I was allowed some food! I started with liquids, then soft solids. I still felt weak but was definitely on the mend. Later I found out that when the surgeon first talked to my wife after the surgery, he told her if I pulled through, I'd feel better than I had in years. Neither my wife nor I realized how close I'd come to my final hours.

I shared my room with another fellow. He had an eye injury that resulted in the loss of light vision in one eye. The doctors would come around and check to see if he improved. As his hospital stay lengthened though, his physical condition seemed to worsen. His apparent deterioration was psychological, and his eye didn't recover. It was a strange situation. I had the dangerous condition that threatened my life and I progressed each day. Other than his eye, he was in good physical condition when he arrived then went downhill each day.

I was pretty weak when I went home. At first, I was able to walk across a room and that was about it. I wasn't allowed to drive or lift more than 15 pounds. My life involved taking walks, eating, and sleep. The doctors all agreed that Crohn's disease caused this near catastrophe for me. I often wondered about the association between bowel disease and AS.

I also knew there would be a time in the future when I would live up to the commitment that I made in my prayers. But my problems had not gone away. They were just at a better level. For the long run, I was not out of trouble yet.

Lessons Learned

Each individual has a responsibility for their own well-being. I for one never wanted to put total reliance of my health on physicians. So, with that in mind, I knew I needed to develop a plan. The idea that there was no cure for Crohn's disease left me facing a future of difficulties that I didn't want. It seemed like facing a life sentence.

I had survived the crash but was on a lot of medications. I ate lots of foods with no diet restrictions. I was really hungry, eating meals with large portions and loading up on high calorie snacks. I ate over a pound of cookies a day. I gained a pound or more of weight each day for a while even though my symptoms were still there but diminished.

On one of my follow-up visits with the surgeon, I asked if there was anything I could do to help myself with diet. He hesitated but did say that doctors sometimes suggest removing dairy-containing products. I immediately set about to do this.

Eliminating milk and cheese was easy. Dairy products are used in so many foods, so for the first time, we started to read labels. I eliminated dairy for about six months to give it a chance to see if it would help. My symptoms didn't improve during this trial, so I did go back on dairy and quit reading the labels.

Over the next year, I went through a period of gaining body weight followed by my weight stabilizing at a weight higher than I had ever attained in my life. I was very encouraged by this! Unfortunately, some symptoms remained. In the second year after the crash, I started losing weight again. This worried me. It was very gradual, but a deterioration started all over again.

I saw my general practitioner and an internist. I had lots of prescriptions to take. Blood tests were routine. In spite of all this attention, I still felt trouble brewing. I feared facing another life-threatening episode unless something changed. I just had no idea what the change involved.

My prayers were to be answered and I have tried to subsequently live up to the commitments that I made. First though, I needed to find a way to regain my health.

So, philosophically, it was ingrained in my mind that there was in fact a way to get better but discovering that challenge that was up to me. What I was looking for was not going to be handed to me on a silver platter. In the maze of information and the maze of life, it was out there for me to find it.

Chapter 6

My Library Research Years

I brainstormed in my mind on how to go forward. My first step then was to start learning more. How best to learn more? I went to the library. I envisioned reading books and technical articles on the subject so that I'd at least become knowledgeable. I needed to find ways to help myself because inside a collision course with disaster lurked. My deterioration was slow. I had some time.

The library was about a 20-minute drive from the house. At this point, it was safe for me to drive again. Within a minute of entering the building, I felt an urgent need for the restroom. Afterwards, I went straight to the card catalog to look up books on my topic and find them on the shelves. Again, the sense of urgency reappeared and I ran quickly to the bathroom.

I checked out some books and went home. Over the next few weeks, the process of studying and learning was underway. Crohn's disease is part of a family of autoimmune diseases called Irritable Bowel Disease (IBD). Both Crohn's disease and Ulcerative Colitis are the major ones. For some unexplained reason, the body's own immune system attacks itself causing distress. There were lists of other autoimmune diseases such as multiple sclerosis in this family of diseases.

I returned to the library for my second visit to return my books and look for some more. Like my first trip there, I felt an immediate need for the restroom. Something about this building was impacting me. I returned my books and checked out several titles, leaving quickly. A month later during my visit, the pattern repeated itself, and continued on for several years of visits later.

Through my readings, I didn't come across anything that pointed to something in the air that might affect people with Crohn's disease. I read books, I read articles in the technical journals. And slowly still, my health deteriorated.

Suppose a person were to go to their doctor and tell him that Crohn's disease symptoms were impacted in a negative way by simply entering a library. My doctor was not interested in this. It was discounted as not important.

My readings and study led me to conclude my doctors were providing me with mainstream treatments. My healthcare needs were taken care of, yet my health was sliding.

I became more knowledgeable but found no inkling of a path to improvement. I needed to change my line of thinking, so I made a shift in the materials I was researching. The mainstream medical books and article reading changed to simply looking for articles and books that gave examples of people like me getting better, regardless of the source.

I was crossing over into the "anecdotal" world. Anecdotes aren't considered reliable information by the mainstream medical world, but then doctors and medicine apparently had little more to offer me anyway. I had nothing to lose.

The question became, where in the library should I look to find this kind of information? I had to live with the physical discomfort of going there and persevere.

My limit there was one hour. Once I left, I started feeling better quickly. On one trip I went into the books relating to allergies. Who knows, maybe I would find something. I had tried the dairy-free diet with no positive result and the mainstream books indicated that foods eaten played no role in Crohn's disease. I did however know my airborne allergies existed, so if nothing else, it might help me with those.

I started thumbing through books to find some stories (anecdotes) about people with digestive system distress (not Crohn's disease) getting better. I read through book after book, picking out the pages that seemed related to it. While I felt I was getting closer, I really had arrived at no direction.

Through sampling of library books, there were a few references that seemed to make a vague tie between food allergy and Crohn's disease. I left the library that day with a title that was referenced in a book and headed straight for a bookstore.

I found the book, *Complete Book of Allergy Control* by Laura J. Stevens there. I polished the book off in two days. Stevens indicated that Crohn's disease may possibly be related to food allergy.[11] She also suggested that a yeast infection can weaken the body's immune system leading to Crohn's disease among others.[12]

After reading this, I concluded there was a glimmer of hope, that there were possibilities. Based on the Stevens book, I was back to the bookstore and found *The Yeast Syndrome* by John Trowbridge, M.D., and Morton Walker, D.P.M.

This book had several case studies where people sick with Crohn's disease got better - significantly better. Early in the book I found the following:

> *"Are you interested in knowing of a safe, effective, tested, legal, non-surgical treatment which can eliminate diarrhea, chronic belly pain, inflammation, ulceration, and malabsorption in your gut, even possibly conditions known as colitis, enteritis, ileitis, or Crohn's disease?"*[13]

My answer to this was an excited yes! What interested me were the case studies sprinkled throughout the book. People with various symptoms were being treated in ways that I'd never heard of before, ways that seemed unorthodox.

My mind stewed over this information. After years and years of being sick, this was the first material that I'd come across that gave me a feeling that there might be a chance, even though small, of getting better. I suppose that my thinking was dominated by emotion but was operating at least in a somewhat logical manner.

In addition to the stories, there was a list of doctors located around the country in the back of the book. One of the doctors was in my city. I could go see him! I could find out if he had something to offer.

I started making inquiries to people I knew about this physician. He had a very good reputation and had graduated from a highly respected medical school. He was a general practitioner. The stories I heard from people were surprising. Multiple people said they'd improve under his care when other doctors had failed. A person I worked closely with had experienced sore throats for about 20 years. He'd been to many doctors for many treatments with little success. He felt he'd been handed a small miracle and gave this doctor stellar marks.

Another person reported that his child had a rather spectacular improvement while under this doctor's care. Although neither of these testimonials related directly to my health challenges, I wanted to believe that maybe he could help me as well.

Without mentioning this doctor by name, I showed my internist the book highlighting some of the stories within. He didn't use the word 'quackery' but it was certainly implied.

One night I was flipping through the television channels and came across a speech by a doctor regarding the treatment of hyperactive children. He reported that when he started practicing medicine, he employed the techniques he was taught in medical school. Unfortunately, he was less than satisfied with the results. He told a story about a hyperactive child given an "upper" which resulted in calming the child, just the opposite of the expected effect.

He also treated hyperactive children by advising their mothers to remove favorite foods from the child's diet. This often resulted in better results than the approaches he'd learned in medical school. Often the foods that were removed from the children's diet were snacks and junk foods. Seeing this helped me to make my decision.

Health-wise, I was still going in the wrong direction, even though I was given treatments people like me should be getting. I decided the risk in going to see this doctor was minimal and made an appointment.

Chapter 7

A New Direction

My first visit to the new doctor didn't go as expected. I didn't even see him. Instead, I saw a nurse whose job was to record my case history. She asked many questions for over an hour to get the information the doctor required. This case history process and the time invested before seeing the doctor was something I had never experienced before. It struck me that it was a good idea. It seemed better than a doctor asking what the current symptoms are and getting a prescription.

My next visit was with Dr. John. He'd read my case history beforehand so he was familiar with my issues. During the discussion, I asked the question that I really wanted an answer to. "Can you help me?" Without hesitation, he responded, "I think I can but I'm not certain." Next, I asked if he had treated Crohn's disease patients successfully. His response was that he had not but had some success with ulcerative colitis.

The thought that he said he might be able to help me was much better than previous experiences. I felt cautiously optimistic.

Dr. John advised me that the standard treatments are designed for the typical or average person. There are people who differ sufficiently from the average such that the standard approaches may not be effective, while for others it may be very effective. He advised that my history of allergies was a good sign that he might be able to help me get better.

His first suggestion was to try an air purifier in my bedroom. He said that a person typically spends 8 or more hours a day there. I rented one from a nearby pharmacy and placed it as he requested very close to the head of the bed. It was kind of noisy and made the room smell funny. I thought maybe this is what a room would smell like with the dust and impurities at reduced levels due to air purification. It's also possible that the unit I used was emitting ozone.

What to do with the multitude of prescriptions I was already taking as recommended by my doctor of internal medicine? Dr. John advised me that I should stay on my previously prescribed medicines.

Risks associated with the new approach I was heading into was a concern. Dr. John quickly said there'd be virtually no risk to me. That was enough for me. I was ready to proceed. I now had a small glimmer of hope that I would get better. My research to this point had offered me no hope. I had to do this. The thought of another crash was too much. I had to find a way.

He started with me as an allergy patient. The good news was that my insurance at the time paid 100% for allergy treatment. On a subsequent visit, I was given skin tests for various substances. My research had mentioned that skin tests are not particularly reliable of food allergies, so I remained skeptical at first. I reacted to many of the substances with strong reactions to potato and soy. Potatoes had long been a favorite of mine that I ate almost every day. Where was the soy from? After reading labels on packaging when I got home, soy is in many food products that I probably ate every day.

I thought back to the television show where the doctor told the mothers to remove their children's favorite food from their diet and favorable responses often followed. Was I heading in this direction? I immediately stopped eating potatoes and any food with soy in it and started feeling a little better.

Another round of testing was prescribed by Dr. John. This time I was sent to a lab for a blood draw. The test used is called the RAST (radio-allegro-sorbent-test). Clinically significant results are scored at 4, 5, or 6 and 6 is the maximum positive result. The first round of these tests resulted in the following:

Corn	6
Egg White	6
Milk	6
Peanut	6
Soy Bean	6
Candida	6
Wheat	4
Cane Sugar	3

Broken down this meant that 75% of substances tested maxed out at 6, and the others were clinically significant (87%).

I looked at these results with mixed feelings. What I didn't know for sure was where we were going with this information. I was starting to get the feeling that I was allergic to the world! Under all those thoughts though were feelings of hope and understanding.

After reviewing these results, Dr. John sent me to get more blood drawn. The results of this 2nd round was as follows:

Pork	6
Apple	5
Broccoli	5
Carrot	5
Chicken	5
Oat	5
Rice	5
Sweet Potato	3
Beef	2
Beet	2

At least there weren't as many 6's this time! To summarize, the checks on 18 substances resulted in 39 % with a maximum score of 6 with 78% clinically significant.

Next there was an evaluation period that consisted of several diets that were used for short periods of time. By diet, I'm not referring to weight loss regimens; rather, foods to eat that would help understand their impact on my symptoms. Yes, a human guinea pig.

One of the diet trials lasted only a few days, but it had a favorable impact on my digestive system. On the 3rd day of this diet which was also the last day, I was required to eat a relatively large amount of sugar. This caused me dizziness. The feeling of dizziness after consuming sugar really impacted me and was totally unexpected. Remember the bag of cookies I ate every day!

Another diet used for a week and a half trial he called the Stone Age Diet. I was asked to keep records of what I ate and how I felt. My symptoms were changing simultaneously to the changing foods eaten. Often, the changes were for the better.

Dr. John next asked me to try a "drop" program. This one I really never understood but the basic idea seemed to be that if a substance is given under the tongue and in the correct quantity, it can in some people turn on and off an allergic reaction to the substance. During the period of time I took the drops, I didn't notice an impact.

As the spring airborne allergy season was arriving, Dr. John prescribed an antihistamine to help deal with sinus issues. He also suggested that the antihistamine if taken all year around might have a favorable impact on my digestive system distresses.

There is some logic for using the antihistamine and the air purifier. When a person is under bombardment from particles in the air resulting in an allergic reaction, the body's defenses mobilize to fight the intruders. While this is going on, I theorized that the body might be in a weaker condition in an area such as the digestive system.

After about two months with Dr. John, I was off potatoes and soy on the food side and was using an air purifier and an antihistamine on the allergy front. My health was improving for the first time in 15 years.

I was still having my monthly appointments with the doctor of internal medicine. At that two-month mark he took me off of anti-inflammatory drugs that I'd been on to manage the pain associated with AS. Before, I could not get along at all without it, and still had some residual pain. With one pill gone, I remained on all the others. While they really didn't help me much, I decided that I would stay on them until the doctor that prescribed them advised me to stop.

5-Day Rotation Diet

The third month into seeing Dr. John, he made his major recommendation for my treatment going forward. He told me that he had considered a 4-day and a 5-day rotation diet for me to use. He said the 5-day rotation diet plan was tougher but given my physical condition, that is what I needed.

I was venturing into new territory. In my wildest imagination I had never dreamed that the treatment I would be given would be a change of what I was eating. I thought up to this point that one goes to a doctor to get a prescription.

Dr. John told me to expect my weight to drop at first, maybe around 10 pounds. With my long history of struggling to maintain body weight, this was definitely not what I wanted to hear.

When I recovered from the crash, my weight had increased to a new high for me. Over the succeeding six years, 14 pounds were gradually lost. I was already heading in the wrong direction in terms of weight.

He did say the risk was low and progress was seen. Who knows, it sure seemed worth trying as nothing had really helped me over the last 15 years. The food rotation plan that Dr. John presented to me is found in Figure 7-1.

The proposed diet is a real WYSIWIG (what you see is what you get). To follow the diet, I wasn't allowed to eat anything at all that was not listed on this chart.

For example, on day 1 for breakfast I could have 2 eggs, a bowl of cream of wheat (nothing on it) and apple juice (unsweetened) to drink. For lunch, I could have a plain chicken breast (no seasonings), plain asparagus, and an apple along with apple juice. Pecans are an option on day 1 and can be used as a snack.

If you look through a given day, foods on the list can be chosen and that item constitutes a meal menu item. With this approach, my body experienced a significant reduction in total number of ingredients in a meal. It was pretty common for a meal to have 5 items and also 5 total ingredients of those items combined.

To help myself at the time with ideas for recipes for a rotation diet, I purchased and referred to frequently the book, *If This Is Tuesday, It Must Be Chicken, or How to Rotate Your Food for Better Health* by Natalie Golos and Frances Golos Golbitz.[14] Eating this way was very different and challenging.

FIVE DAY ROTATION DIET					
FOOD TYPE	DAY #1	DAY #2	DAY #3	DAY #4	DAY #5
Meat	Chicken Eggs Pheasant	Lamb Pork Venison	Fish Duck	Turkey Rabbit Crab Shrimp Oysters Lobster	Beef
Vegetable	Lettuce Onion Asparagus Artichoke	Carrots Celery Parsley Parsnips	Spinach Beets Chard Tomato Potato (white)	Yams Legumes: Peas G. Beans Soybean Cucumber Squash	Cabbage Broccoli Brussels Sprout Turnips Radish Corn
Fruit	Apple Pear	Lemon Grapefruit Orange Tangerine	Banana Berries Raspberry Strawberry Blackberry	Canteloupe Pineapple Grape Raisins Coconut	Apricot Plum Prune Peaches Nectarine
Cereals/Starch	Wheat Flour	Tapioca Oats	Arrowroot Flour Potato Starch	Rice Rice Flour	Cornstarch Oats
Beverage	Apple Juice Mate Tea	Orange Juice (fresh) Grapefruit Juice Sassafras Tea	Tomato Juice	Grape Juice	Rose Hips Tea Milk
Nuts	Pecan Walnut	Cashew	Brazil Nut	Peanut Filbert	Almond
Oil	Sunflower	Sesame	Safflower Avacado	Peanut Soy	Olive Corn
Sweetener	Cane Sugar	Honey	Beet Sugar	Date Sugar Artificial Sweetener	Maple Syrup Karo
NOTE WELL: Buckwheat is not related to the wheat family and may be used on another day as cereal.					

Figure 7-1. Starting point for a five-day rotation diet plan.

Along with the diet, I was instructed to keep data on how I felt each day and also the level of my symptoms. Dr. John told me that as I would be eating food in a repetitive pattern, a symptom or symptoms might occur which followed the pattern of the food. Should that happen, I was by trial and error to remove something from the diet until the culprit was found.

I took the diet sheet home and showed it to my family. It was not looked upon with great favor. No one in the family wanted to join me in eating this way. We decided the approach to take would be for me to eat separate meals. I was desperate, so I was quite willing to do this. I also knew that I would need to be very disciplined.

We worked out a plan so that I could be on this program 100% of the time. My "food" day would start at dinner and end at lunch the next day. Consecutive dinners, breakfasts, and lunches were from the same rotation diet. This allowed me to use dinner leftovers for lunch the following day. I would take the leftover meal to work and reheat the food in the microwave. This made following the diet a lot easier.

The rotation diet plan required eating foods only on the allowed day, once every five days. For example, milk occurs once in the rotation and is not eaten again for five days. This required some discipline as it doesn't allow eating snacks and other fun foods during that day. Also required to do this diet was reading the labels of food items. Every single one.

Reading the labels got to be very interesting yet challenging. Many grocery items were exempt from the diet because the ingredients included items from more than one diet day. I was advised to avoid artificial ingredients and preservatives. This left very few grocery items that I could use.

Fresh fruit and vegetables were good as well as the frozen variety. Canned foods could only be used selectively.

My menu featured foods that I had never before eaten in my life and in some cases, just plain did not want. When faced with the possibility of getting better, eating foods I didn't like seemed to be the lesser of two evils. If I could find answers to my health issues from the gut, so be it.

The diet needed to be followed religiously. The most difficult challenges would be when I was away from home, like business trips or visiting family in another city. The latter was easiest to deal with. My mother really embraced the diet and would fix me foods according to the plan when I called ahead. I did the best I could on business trips. This sometimes meant eating according to the plan for that particular day, but not ordering as much food as I would have liked due to it not being available at the restaurant.

Within days after going on the diet, I started feeling better than I had in years. The numbers on the chart I kept were headed in the right direction. Symptoms such as chills cleared up. I'd been warned of potential weight loss and that happened. While I was feeling much, much better, my weight was going down. I eventually lost 13 pounds.

I'd been using statistics as part of my job for a number of years. The chart I developed enabled me to interpret the data quickly and easily. Early in the program, I noticed a blip on the chart every time Day 3 rolled around. I called the doctor's office and was advised to start trial and error tests to find the offending food.

I removed each item one at a time when Day 3 came around. Each evaluation took five days as I had to wait five days to remove that item to gauge any reaction to it, and then proceed on with another food. I tried all the foods on the days the blip showed up on the chart. Initially, I found no culprit. I was pretty puzzled. Then it dawned on me that the problem food might actually be food I'd eaten the day before the symptoms showed up. I started one-by-one removing the items from the prior day and hit the jackpot. It was the orange juice. I removed that from day #2 and the blip disappeared.

I switched to grapefruit and grapefruit juice, then the symptoms - while still there but at a lower level, reduced. I eventually dropped citrus products entirely from the diet. I substituted papaya juice based on a recommendation from the doctor's staff. I didn't care for papaya juice at all, but could live with it due to making progress. Later through a similar process I found that banana was causing similar symptoms.

Before I started the 5-day rotation plan, I eliminated soy and soy products. I realized that prior to changing the way I ate, I'd been eating problem foods all along every single day.

My research told me the current logic is that diet bears no relation to Crohn's disease. I clearly know that's not correct. A person like me with bowel disease does react to the foods they eat, however, doesn't react to all foods in equal ways. Some foods can lead to symptoms and some do not. Eating in a highly structured way showed proof to me.

I tried years earlier to eliminate dairy and it had no effect. Eliminating one variable at a time is a slow process that may not reveal a result, as in my case, because of multiple food sensitivities. The stringent 5-day plan afforded me to diagnose each one more simply.

My weight loss needed to be addressed. Dr. John's office made arrangements for me to see a nutritionist their office worked with. We met several times and she evaluated my program and concurred with the doctor's view that I was on the right track. She did suggest that I start eating nuts to try to get more calories. Nuts have 160 to 200 calories per ounce. I quickly saw that it was not going to take many nuts to make an impact on my caloric intake.

We bought cashews, peanuts, Brazil nuts, pecans, walnuts, and almonds. I went on a nut rotation that lined up with the foods I was eating. This brought the weight loss to a halt and gradually my weight started to go up.

By now, I'd been on the rotation diet plan for over 6 months. I was gaining weight. My level of digestive system distress continued to be better than it had been in many years and my other symptoms were trending in the right direction.

During this time, I continued to see my internist who had no knowledge of what I was doing regarding diet. He hinted at the outset that this approach might be quackery, so I saw no need to tell him.

Over time, he gradually reduced the number and quantity of medications. As he saw my symptoms decrease and my weight increase, he took the appropriate action. After one of my visits, he reached the point of ending my last medication outside of using an antihistamine occasionally.

I was pretty much prescription free! This doctor told me that the medications that he'd given me had finally "kicked in." Now stop and think about this. If you were a doctor, would you really believe that the effect of a medicine kicked in after six years bringing forth the improvement? It would have been much better for him to suggest that unknown factors had led to the improvement.

After I was off the medications, I never went back to see him. I believe he was conscientiously trying to help me, but the tools he'd been taught were ineffective for me. He followed the mainstream playbook for cases like mine – no fault to him. The truth was that the medications weren't known to be particularly effective, so the results I experienced were not unusual.

After I had been eating without exception to the rotation diet plan, Dr. John suggested that I do a test by eating a small amount of something outside the diet schedule and see what would happen. This really raised my curiosity.

I ate a small amount of one food item in violation of the plan. Nothing happened. The next day was a different matter. I experienced a surge of digestive distress. I felt horrible that whole day. The next day was better. It took three days for me to get back to my normal state of well-being. I waited a month or so and tried it again with another food item. Same result.

When there's a problem where you can turn the problem off and on, it's thought that the root cause has been found. This concept is straight out of textbooks associated with the quality assurance profession in manufacturing.

The soreness in my neck due to AS simultaneously improved to the point that it became a non-issue and my digestive system was working well (only mild symptoms).

My health was now much better than it had been. I felt pretty good. Changing the foods had not shown up in any of the research as a positive way to get improvement. In fact, it was discouraged. Had this diet been suggested to me years earlier, a lot of suffering and distress would've been alleviated.

Chapter 8

Major Problem Results in New Insight

It was the middle of winter during my first year on the diet. At my office, some of the employees started to experience nose bleeds and sore throats. At first it was a few people, but each day the numbers increased. The company had two office complexes - one on the north side of the factory and one on the south. The north office employees and the factory employees were unaffected. It was the south office employees only.

There was no obvious reason we could see that would indicate the cause. The environment seemed quite normal. The company had employee meetings to assure everyone they were trying to determine what was causing it. Several days went by and the ill employees started becoming absent, and more were becoming ill. The majority of employees were fine though.

I started to experience soreness in my neck again. Was my AS coming back?

After a few days, I couldn't drive. Additionally, my right hip and left foot started to hurt as well. Each day these symptoms became worse.

I told management what was happening to me. In return, I received some peculiar looks. My symptoms didn't match what other people were experiencing. Another day went by and I asked to be moved to the north complex. This could not continue. They said they'd consider my request. Absenteeism was on the rise and morale was low.

Then they called us in for a meeting the next day and advised that management had contracted with a company to sample and analyze the air in the offices. The company came in very quickly, gathered their samples, and took them back to their lab for analysis. The next day the results of the study came in.

Sulfur dioxide was the culprit. Adjacent to the south office complex was a boiler. The boiler had a malfunction which had not been detected and sulfur dioxide was leaking into the south office. Sulfur dioxide is an odorless colorless poisonous gas. We couldn't smell it or see any indication of it. The boiler was shut down immediately.

I was pretty sore and uncomfortable by then. I called Dr. John's office and asked for a recommendation to deal with this issue. He told me to take Vitamin B12 under my tongue. I followed the suggestion and was much better in a short time. I returned to normal in a few days.

This incident was really important for me. I experienced a 'referred' symptom, which means the symptom was caused by a source outside of where a symptom occurs. This incident reminded me of the discomfort I felt at the library.

Through this episode of sulfur dioxide exposure, there were quite a few people who were unaffected. They went about their work duties as if there were no issue. Here is a case where a number of people were exposed to a poisonous gas, yet some experienced no symptoms. This is a really important concept. People can be experiencing a problem, but for some reason, had a higher tolerance for this poisonous gas.

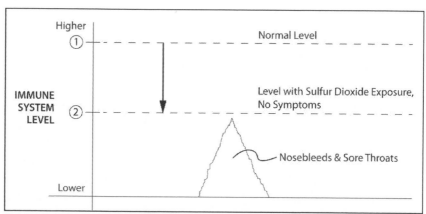

Figure 8-1. Exposure to sulfur dioxide gas with no symptoms.

Referring to Figure 8-1, let's suppose that the immune system of a person is normally operating at Level 1. With the exposure to the poisonous gas, the immune system goes into action and some of that precious resource is used and is drawn down to Level 2. If the mountain in the diagram represents symptoms such as nose bleeds and sore throats, one can see that Level 2 is not low enough for the onset of symptoms. Now let's consider the case where symptoms are present in a person with the same sulfur dioxide gas exposure.

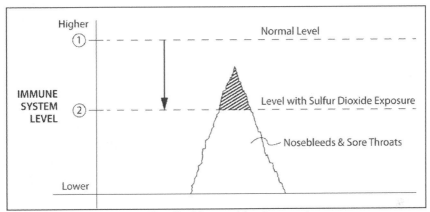

Figure 8-2. Exposure to sulfur dioxide resulting in symptoms.

The immune system level has gone down to the point that the threshold for symptoms has been crossed. If other demands are placed on the body or the sulfur dioxide level increases, symptoms can be expected to increase.

Referring to Figure 8-2, the diagram was changed only in the height of the mountain or the sensitivity of a person to breathing the poisonous gas. In this case, the person suffers symptoms.

Now if we assume the amount of sulfur dioxide gas were to increase, then the dashed line representing the immune system would go further down the chart and the symptoms would increase in intensity (as represented by the shaded area in Figure 8-2). As the amount of the gas in the air becomes more and more, the immune system is used up at the point that it's no longer able to contain health issues. At this point is when illness, injuries, or even death can occur.

Exposure to sulfur dioxide at a level that causes illness (Figure 8-2) in some individuals is also bad for those not suffering ill effects (Figure 8-1). Though not everyone showed symptoms, everyone involved was being poisoned by this pollutant.

An example of another air pollutant is radon. It's found in high concentrations in some geographic locations and sometimes in some common places such as in houses, particularly in basements. Radon is also odorless and colorless.

We have no way of knowing it's present without testing for it. Radon is the second leading cause of lung cancer in the United States, second only to smoking tobacco.

According to the American Cancer Society:

"Cigarette smoking is by far the most common cause of lung cancer in the United States, but radon is the second leading cause. Scientists estimate that about 20,000 lung cancer deaths per year are related to radon."[15]

People can experience years of exposure to high levels of radon and not realize it's an issue. Not everyone who experiences significant long-term radon exposure will get lung cancer, but the incidence rate clearly goes up with exposure. This is a time-delay type of process.

Everything seems fine for years and then some incur unexpected lung cancer. People can go through many years of exposure considered unacceptable and not realize it. For some poisonous gases such as sulfur dioxide and radon, the same exposure can result in a range from no symptoms to significant health issues in different people. All people do not react the same way to the same problem.

While it may seem like a quantum leap, one could make a case that the same appears to be true for foods that we eat. Some people can eat foods and apparently suffer no impact while others like me can eat the same thing and be extremely sick.

For example, when I tested my rotation plan diet by eating something not on the list, I chose to eat some corn - just a small dish. The next day I felt awful and it took three days to recover.

Now I was thinking about why the rotation diet was helping me so much. I was feeling lots better - not yet to 100% but pretty good. The textbooks for rotation diets talk about them being good for people with food sensitivities or allergies.

The food rotation plan did a couple of things: eliminated a number of problem foods from my diet, and since getting healthier, my immune system was under a greatly reduced load and therefore much more effective.

It was clear to me that exposure to some poisonous gases could lead to some people being symptom free while others became ill. The difference depends to some extent on the level of an individual's immune system. A person with an immune system operating at a very high healthy level could withstand a higher exposure to a toxin such as sulfur dioxide before the onset of symptoms as compared to a person whose immune system is already weakened. This is a big leap as well but it could be that some foods we ingest are causing a similar impact.

Before I went on the rotation plan, I thought that all foods bothered me, but I found out that wasn't true. Not all foods impacted me equally nor do I believe that foods impact people in the same way. At the time, when I ate corn, big distresses occurred for me. Most people would have eaten the corn and not experienced a problem. Like the odorless, colorless sulfur dioxide, I began to wonder if corn is bad for everyone. Most would assume that the problem was on my end since I didn't tolerate corn very well. While most think corn is a good, healthy food, is it really?

While I have just singled out corn, I began to realize that the rotation diet plan that was being a huge help to my well-being had also eliminated many items and reduced quantities of others. I was eating more vegetables, more variety of meats, and more fruits. I was eating no candies or junk foods. Long a staple of my diet, potatoes were out.

The rotation food plan not only put me on a repeating cycle on terms of what I was eating, but what I was eating changed greatly. Making more than one change at a time in foods eaten resulted in what is called confounding. In other words, I could not clearly determine what was affecting the changes my body was experiencing. I know for sure that using the approach of changing one food at a time would likely never have gotten me to the point of getting better. I was better because I had changed a whole lot of foods all at once.

Many books are available on rotation diet plans. They've been around for many years and found to be useful. What is believed is that rotation diets raise the level of the immune system. As in Figures 8-1 & 8-2, the higher the immune system level, the less likely for symptoms. I suspect that not many mainstream doctors use rotation diet plans nor even know what they are.

People affected by some foods may exhibit no short-term symptoms. In my case, I had more foods that negatively impacted me that compromised my immune system to such an extent that I displayed a multitude of symptoms. The healthy people around me appeared to be able to eat most anything with no issues or minimal issues. I guess this meant I was still abnormal.

The mainstream medical community really doesn't have a direct measure of the immune system. Doctors can base their view, on an indirect basis, on case histories and some blood tests that give limited information on this subject.

All I really knew at this point was my weight was going up with little digestive distress, and I was medication free outside of the antihistamine. Things were looking brighter.

Chapter 9

Airborne Allergens

I followed the 5-day rotation food plan for the next several years and the dramatic relief from the digestive distress continued. I gained weight to the point that new, larger clothes were needed. I was no longer severely underweight. My overall health and well-being rose to new levels and yet I was almost medication free.

Dr. John had me take an antihistamine all year around at first. He thought it would help as the spring season arrived. I dutifully took the one remaining prescription as all others had been discontinued by my other doctor.

What happened over the next few years was to me nothing short of amazing. Having severe symptoms from spring-to-frost airborne allergens for me was the norm. This started to change and change for the better.

The first year on the antihistamine and the food rotation plan was a little better in terms of symptoms relating to the airborne allergens. That was something very good, but it was not a lot different. It could have just been a more favorable year in terms of what was in the air. The second year was even better. This was starting to look like a trend. Then the third year rolled around and that year was even better yet. Wow!

Over several years, my symptoms relating to airborne allergens cleared up and I was able, under Dr. John's direction, to stop using the antihistamine altogether.

For the first time in many years, I was medication free and feeling the best I had in years. My chronic hay fever and asthmatic symptoms were relieved and my severe Crohn's disease was under control. This had to be a miracle. Prayers had been answered.

Over the years, I've talked to a number of people complaining about airborne allergens. In conversations, I mentioned having pretty significant spring-to-frost airborne allergen issues leading in some cases to pneumonia in the fall season. They would invariably ask what I had done that made a difference. I told them that I cleared my symptoms by changing what I ate. Invariably, the expression on their face was disbelief. It just didn't make sense to them. How can food eaten relate to sinus and asthmatic conditions?

Like the exposure to sulfur dioxide previously discussed, airborne allergens result in symptoms for some people. It's also true that many in the population are exposed to airborne allergens and exhibit no symptoms.

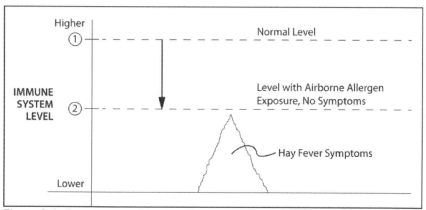

Figure 9-1. Exposure to airborne allergens such as pollens with no symptoms exhibited.

Through the hay fever season each year, there are quite a few people who are unaffected. They go about their daily lives with no symptoms. Figure 9-1 shows the case where a person is exposed to airborne allergens and exhibits no symptoms. The human body is impacted by this and the immune system reacts and as is the case for many people, no symptoms occur. It's important to note that the immune system is impacted even though there are no outward symptoms.

The entire population in a region is exposed to airborne allergens simultaneously. Some do exhibit symptoms at various levels. Figure 9-2 shows the case where a person's immune system reaction is insufficient to avoid symptoms such as a runny nose and watery eyes. Compared to Figure 9-1, the diagram was changed only in the height of the mountain or the sensitivity of a person to airborne allergens.

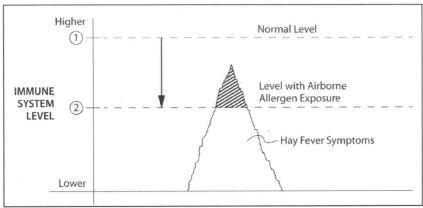

Figure 9-2. Exposure to airborne allergens such as pollens in symptoms.

If the amount of airborne allergens were to increase, then the dashed line representing the immune system would go further down the chart and the symptoms would increase in intensity (as represented by the shaded area in Figure 9-2). As the amount of airborne allergens decreases, such as after the first hard frost in colder climates, the immune system is less taxed. The immune system then operates at a higher level while simultaneously the symptoms clear up for the season.

For many years, my body was under siege by both Crohn's disease and airborne allergens. It's reasonable to think that my immune resources were drained. When I changed my foods, I got relief in terms of Crohn's disease symptoms. The load on my immune system decreased which left more of this precious resource to deal with hay fever symptoms. The result being is that both my Crohn's disease symptoms and hay fever symptoms improved as a result of the same root cause.

The foods I'd been eating over many years were the culprit. I had the hay fever symptoms for many years prior to the onset of Crohn's disease symptoms. I think that when I made a major change to my food choices, it became apparent that I had uncovered the reason my body was experiencing airborne allergens symptoms.

As the internet was becoming more popular, I became involved in a group of people online that had digestive distresses. I tried to tell them my story of getting better. That really went nowhere. I wasn't able to convince anyone to try changing their food. I did however find that the digestive distresses of the folks worsened in the spring and the fall. These people were often suffering from worsening digestive distress during the prime airborne allergen seasons. I was starting to understand that there was a connection. Bowel disease symptoms could vary somewhat with the seasons.

George was someone who I knew and had suffered from bowel disease for years. I remember his wife telling the story of her husband being hospitalized four consecutive years in the month of August for Crohn's disease. She thought that was quite a coincidence. I was taking this story in and knew this was very unlikely a coincidence. I immediately suspected that George's symptoms were worsening because of the load on his body from airborne allergens during the hay fever season. He wasn't experiencing hay fever symptoms, so he didn't grasp the connection. The symptom's expression in George to airborne allergens was an increase in the severity of his digestive symptoms to the point of hospitalization. One does not need to be an expert in statistics to figure out that hospitalizations four years in a row in the same month is very unlikely due to chance.

Like the folks online that I'd interacted with, I shared my view of George's "August" phenomena. Everyone I suggested the idea to was polite and nice, but it was obvious my words were met with more than skepticism.

I should mention here that my first operation for Crohn's disease also occurred in the month of August. That was not a coincidence either in my view.

The online group turned out to be a close-knit group of people. I made absolutely no headway in convincing anyone of the possibilities of improved health through diet though. The message from the doctors that diet had no impact was ringing through loud and clear to these people scattered about the country.

Their doctors were telling them all the same story which coincided with what I had found in my library research. This was the mainstream mantra. Food is not the issue. The body is malfunctioning due to an autoimmune disease. Here I was trying to help people, getting nowhere in that quest. I was better and the people I was interacting with were not moved at all.

It was through this group that I found out about the book, *Food and the Gut Reaction* by Elaine Gottschall.[16] A person in the group claiming to be Dr. Smith in Pennsylvania told folks he had Crohn's disease and used this book to recover. He said that he kept copies of this book at his office to make it available to patients. "Smith" turned out to be a bogus name but the book itself was very real.

Finding Elaine Gottschall's book proved to be really important. I thought I'd found the only way to improve my bowel disease with diet. Now there was a lead to another potential diet. The book had been published in Canada and had some success there. It was little known in the United States. I ordered a copy and wanted to study her diet and compare it to what I was doing with the rotation plan.

In retrospect, I learned some important concepts by going through my diet changes. The human body takes time to make adjustments for changes in inputs in the environment such as ingesting different foods. Not all human's internal processes adjust at the same rate in terms of symptoms. There was relief in a matter of days for digestive-related symptoms and it took several years of trending improvement for the airborne allergen symptoms.

Since it took several years for the hay fever to clear up, my body was still changing and adjusting to the new way of eating. It was a process in the gut that the body needed to go through.

Simultaneous with the improvement in Crohn's symptoms and sinus related issues, my asthma cleared up as well. The periods of difficulty with breathing went away. The issue that led to my early exit from the Army was gone.

Chapter 10

Understanding the Specific Carbohydrate Diet

Gottschall's book did mention it could help people with Crohn's disease and other bowel disorders. Her first book, *Food and the Gut Reaction.* is now out of print, is part text and part recipes. I called Elaine Gottschall on the phone introducing myself, and she graciously talked to me on the subject of the Specific Carbohydrate Diet discussed in her book. She told me her diet was developed by Sydney V. Haas, M.D. who initially was looking for a cure for celiac disease. His studies were documented in the book, *Management of Celiac Disease.*[17] He later applied the diet to various other bowel diseases with success. Elaine told me that this was the breakthrough diet for celiac disease and actually preceded the less effective gluten free diet.

I read both of these books. When she brought the book to the United States from Canada, she gave it an update, a cover change and a new title. It was now called *Breaking the Vicious Cycle: Intestinal Health Through Diet.* I continued to discuss the diet over time with Elaine by phone. She knew that people who used the rotation plans like the one I used experienced success, but felt the Haas diet was a better approach.

Her credentials impressed me. She'd gone to college to major in the biological sciences at the age of 48 leading her to eventually attain a bachelor and master's degree. She was invited to work on a PhD but decided instead to take what she'd learned and get the information out to the public.

I was doing pretty well on the rotation plan. I considered changing to the Specific Carbohydrate Diet but decided against it. I did, however, continue to read and learned from it if for nothing else than to have a back-up plan should it ever be needed.

The diet presented in the book was very different from the food rotation plan that I was on. It looked like it would actually be easier to do. It had a list of what to do and what not to do, but unlike the rotation plan, there was no rigid structure to when foods are eaten.

An important idea that I learned from Elaine was about sugar. She called the single sugar (monosaccharide) one that will "require no further splitting in order to be transported from the intestine into the blood stream."[18] These single sugars are allowed in the diet and include many fruits, honey, and very ripe bananas.

Going Bananas

The idea of very ripe bananas being an allowed food caused me to pause given my past experience. All of my life I was taught to eat fresh bananas - the bright yellow ones. Cut out any brown spots. The really ripe bananas were used in baking for banana bread. I did some reading about bananas.

I found that fresh (green or yellow) bananas contain starch. Starch is a polysaccharide and consists of molecules of monosaccharides bonded together. The digestive process has to break down these bonds so the sugar can be digested. As the banana ages, a chemical process occurs and the starch changes to single sugars which are more easily digested.

What I was learning from Elaine was that a person like me with bowel disease should eat easier-to-digest foods. That sounded pretty logical.

Not allowed on the diet are disaccharides which are often called double sugars - two single sugars bonded together. Foods containing disaccharides include milk, ice cream, maple syrup, chocolate, and table sugar. Sugars with more than two single sugars bonded together such as corn, rice, and pasta are also not allowed.

Elaine also tells us that vegetables that contain more amylose than amylopectin starch (both polysaccharides) are more easily digested.[19] So many vegetables are allowed, but some popular ones are not, such as white and sweet potatoes.

I have provided a partial list of allowed and not allowed foods in APPENDIX A. If you look through the list you'll find many meats, fruits, nuts, and vegetables are allowed. The homemade yogurt, the recipe I've included in APPENDIX B, is essentially lactose free with lactose being a disaccharide.

APPENDIX A is a partial list of foods that are not allowed. Here you'll find some of the foods already mentioned, but in addition, she excludes many of those ingredients found in processed foods as well as all grain-containing foods.

Many lists of foods allowed and not allowed can be found on the internet. I highly suspect that the original source for most of allowed/not allowed lists out there are from Elaine Gottschall herself. She would be very pleased to see that her legacy continued on after her death in 2005, and that the information she provided is much more readily available.

We have all heard the term balanced diet. It is an idea that is not well defined. It does, however, imply that we should eat a variety of foods. If one goes to 10 different sources, one will find 10 different thoughts on what is a balanced diet. Eating a variety of foods offers the opportunity for the body to receive the various vitamins, minerals, and nutrients the body needs. Eating a narrow choice of foods also brings with it an increased opportunity the body will be deprived of something(s) needed.

Eating too much of an item is not eating in a balanced way. Some people consume large amounts of soda pop in a day. Alcoholics drink too much to the detriment of their health and well-being. Chocoholics really like their chocolate, but too much of a good thing can lead to undesirable consequences.

For example, I know some people that eat large amounts of nuts. Nuts are thought by many to be a healthy food and they are allowed on the Specific Carbohydrate Diet. However, in large concentrations nuts can be a problem.

Nuts contain high amounts of oxalates compared to other foods. Oxalates coming from foods can lead to the formation of kidney stones; in some cases, kidney damage. Approximately 75% of kidney stones are made up of calcium oxalate with both the calcium and the oxalate coming from diet. When a person has a kidney stone, it is common for doctors to provide patients with information about foods and their oxalate content hoping the patient will make changes to minimize kidney stones in the future.

There is potentially and even more dire consequence from eating high levels of oxalate laden foods. Those with bowel disease are part of the population that has a number of people with shortened intestines. Doctors cut out diseased bowel tissue and reconnect what remains. A person with a shortened bowel is more susceptible to a disorder called secondary hyperoxaluria than the normal population. The body does not process the oxalate as well in a person with a shortened bowel as compared to a person with natural bowel length. Secondary hyperoxaluria can lead to kidney failure. An additional population that is known to have an increased risk for secondary hyperoxaluria is bariatric patients who've had bowel shortening surgery to help in reducing body weight. A person with secondary hyperoxaluria who also eats foods with high oxalate levels really increases the risk of kidney stones and kidney damage.

I think most of us realize that eating too much of most anything over a long period of time is not good. This remains true for the Specific Carbohydrate Diet. My example is nuts as the Specific Carbohydrate Diet will typically lead to increased nut consumption used in baking and for snacks. There are other examples as well where very high consumption levels of what are thought to be healthy foods are actually unhealthy. In other words, extremes are to be avoided.

Chapter 11

Finding the Answer

Within a couple of years of reading the Gottschall book, while still eating according to the rotation diet plan, I started to experience a skin condition. Spots at first started showing up on my arms. It continued to spread on my arms and my forehead. I needed to scratch the affected areas, so off to the family doctor I went.

He took a look at the conditions on my skin and pulled a reference book off the shelf. The book included pictures. He thumbed through it and found the one he was looking for. He asked me if I thought the picture matched the lesions on my skin. I agreed that it did.

The doctor said the treatment was to take one pill a day of a particular medication for two weeks and then the skin condition should clear up. He wrote the prescription and told me to come back for an appointment after all the pills had been taken.

I took the prescribed pills as instructed. The result was no result. The condition gradually worsened. The itching increased and I became more and more uncomfortable. I went for the two-week visit.

He took one look and referred me to see a dermatologist. He recommended one in the larger city nearby, so the appointment was made. He assured me this doctor was highly regarded in dermatology practice.

At my first appointment, the dermatologist took one look at my skin and without hesitation said I needed to take the regimen of one pill a day for 14 days. I advised him that I'd already done that and it didn't work. He was adamant that I follow his advice and felt this was the correct approach. I did the same treatment the second time.

After completing the two weeks of medication, I returned for the follow-up appointment. The condition was actually slightly worse. It was spreading and itching more. It almost drove me mad. I had monthly appointments with this dermatologist for the next year. He had me take a steroid pill and use a steroid cream on the skin itself. After a year of visits and treatment, there was no improvement in the condition although the steroid cream did give some relief from the itching.

At the end of the year, I point blank asked the dermatologist if he thought he could help me given the lack of results over the last year. He recommended that I take the two-week regimen of pills for the third time. After I was on the pills for several days, I should call him with the results. I agreed.

I was several days into taking the pills again with the same result as the two times before. I called him and shared the outcome. He then advised me he couldn't help me. I thanked him for his efforts but needed a new plan. I decided to go back to my family doctor and see if he had any more thoughts on this. The family doctor, surprised by the dermatologist's words, didn't have any new direction for me. He did suggest that I consider making a change in the carbohydrates I was eating. That one came out of left field!

I went home and gave a lot of thought in trying his suggestion. Then it dawned on me. My back up plan if anything went wrong was to use the Specific Carbohydrate Diet. This diet does in fact remove some carbohydrates. This was something I could try.

Making a major change to a diet is no small order. A couple of weeks was needed to plan the change. Different foods were required and some foods on hand were no longer needed. The day came and the switchover began. This was a big and scary move. I certainly was afraid that the symptoms might come back with a vengeance. But I felt I could always return to the rotation food plan if it didn't work. I started the diet and by the third day, my skin condition made a slight improvement. The digestive system held steady. So far so good.

Over the next three months, the skin condition gradually cleared up - gone like it had never been there. My Crohn's disease also was held at bay, no better and no worse. I was again feeling well and was in no need of medications. Success!

Over the next several years on the Specific Carbohydrate Diet, my health was very good. I continued to be free of the spring-to-frost hay fever symptoms, no asthmatic symptoms, the skin was fine, and the digestive processes were functioning well.

I learned a lot through this experience. I was surprised to find that my skin condition could be treated by adjusting my diet. I was very surprised to find a second diet that favorably impacted my Crohn's disease. I also thought of my family doctor making the suggestion to change carbohydrates in the diet and how all that came together. I still to this day wonder how he came up with the idea.

I still attended support group meetings and started talking about the Specific Carbohydrate Diet and my experience with it. One meeting, I was the featured speaker and made a full presentation on the subject. The group members were very nice, but it was very clear they had no interest in making dietary changes. The point that their symptoms might be relieved or eliminated by digesting certain foods in the gut flew right over their heads. I really felt that it was a failure on my part in my presentation and delivery to gain any measure of interest. I was a little discouraged as I really wanted to find a way to help people.

About three months later, after the support group meeting was over, a lady came up to me and introduced herself. She told me that she worked as a cleaning lady and had attended several support group meetings. She heard my presentation and went out and purchased a copy of Elaine Gottschall's book. She then went on the diet. She now felt so much better she no longer needed to come to our meetings. She'd come at this last meeting just to thank me.

This was an important point in my life as I had helped at least one person with bowel disease to get better!

Chapter 12

Specific Carbohydrate Diet Benefits

When I started the Specific Carbohydrate Diet, my Body Mass Index (BMI) was 17.6 - the limit for underweight being under 18.5. I was skinny, but I'd been thin all my life. Like others with bowel disease that I'd met over the years, it seemed that the more I tried to gain weight, the more frustrated I'd get at failing to achieve the desired result. No matter how much ice cream or potatoes I ate, no weight gain would result.

After a year on the diet, my weight went up and my BMI rose to 22.4. This put me close to the middle of the "normal" range for BMI (range being 18.5 to 24.9). I can personally attest to what Elaine Gottschall was saying about weight normalizing as I followed it.

Before I went on this diet, I was anemic. My iron level had been low for quite a long time. One of my specialists in the past had prescribed an iron supplement. After a couple of days, I didn't feel well. I called the doctor's office and spoke to the nurse to explain that the iron made me feel ill. She told me that since the doctor had prescribed it, I should continue until I was scheduled to see him at my next appointment a month later.

When I saw this specialist, he immediately took me off the iron supplement. My blood test results showed no change. Other than taking iron by infusion which he wanted to avoid, he didn't have many choices.

My next blood test after starting the Specific Carbohydrate Diet showed a spontaneous increase in my iron level. It went up without medication or supplementation. With my iron level up, my energy level made a corresponding improvement.

Being healthy and living a long life aren't the goals of everyone. We often let the short term dominate our lives. What can we experience today, what can we have today? This short-term thinking shows up clearly in the true story that follows below.

A woman named Anne shared this story. Earlier in the year, her daughter Cara went to the hospital emergency room. Her problem had been building for two weeks and finally she'd reached the point where something had to change. Cara had been experiencing frequent bloody bowel movements. This 26-year-old school teacher was weak, scared, and desperately needed help. This emergency room visit turned into a five-day stay.

While in the hospital, Cara was taken off solid food. The idea was to let the intestines rest. She was placed on an IV with fluids including antibiotics and potassium. Lots of tests and evaluations followed resulting in a diagnosis of ulcerative colitis.

Cara was immediately placed on steroids by the doctor in charge. She was to stay away from foods containing fiber and was given some food suggestions. It was recommended that she slowly reintroduce foods back into her diet. She was put on multivitamins and an iron supplement.

The steroids really helped. Over the next month, the dosage of the steroid was gradually reduced until she was weaned off completely. She returned to living her life as normal.

Unfortunately, the improvement was temporary. Her condition gradually deteriorated again. She knew she was still in trouble health wise.

This is where I enter the story. I told Anne that ulcerative colitis is a very serious condition that could eventually lead to the removal of the colon. In addition to the awful symptoms, the irritation leads the person to an elevated cancer risk. We discussed how the Specific Carbohydrate Diet is effective for people with bowel disease and I suggested that she purchase Elaine Gottschall's book. The diet might offer Cara a significant improvement.

Further, I mentioned that doctors try to do their best for patients like Cara but the medications they have in their toolbox were not highly effective. They bring with them a list of possible side effects. It would be in Cara's best interest to change the food she eats to return her bowel to normal function.

I saw Anne several months later who wanted to tell me what had happened in the intervening months.

She did purchase two of Gottschall's books, one copy for herself and one for her daughter. She read the first three chapters to Cara while she laid in bed at her apartment. Both the mom and daughter really tried to understand diet and the effects on the colon, but at this point, no move was made by Cara to change what she was eating.

Cara was sharing a residence with two other women and Anne, fearing her daughter's condition would deteriorate, spoke sternly to the roommates to keep an eye on her. Anne called her daughter frequently and was wrought with worry. A few weeks later, there was another call from the hospital emergency room. Cara's roommates had taken her by car.

Cara's condition was worse this time compared to when she was admitted earlier. The doctors reported that tests showed the colon 90% inflamed on this occasion and she remained in the hospital for seven days. She was given another IV, the same as before, containing potassium and antibiotics. Many tests were made. She was quickly put back on steroids and the iron supplement was stopped. The doctors felt that her intestines couldn't handle it.

They started Cara on Humira injections, this being a very significant medicine with potentially serious side effects. It was suggested that it would take about 2 weeks for this anti-inflammatory to start working. For the short term, Cara moved back home with mom and dad. She wanted a lifestyle change and felt she needed more help in understanding her illness to live.

After moving back home, Anne and Cara worked together and Cara followed the carbohydrate diet with the full support of her mother. They worked hard at it and eliminated all grains, ensured all food groups were eaten each day, and processed foods eliminated. The diarrhea stopped all together and normal frequency for bowel movements returned for the first time since all this had started. Anne told me she felt they were making real headway.

Anne and Cara eventually found out that if Cara followed the diet 100%, she would go into remission. When she departed from the diet, the symptoms would return.

Wanting the Best of Both Worlds

Anne told me that Cara wants to eat a "normal" diet. She wanted to be like her friends. So what she actually did was eat somewhere in between the Specific Carbohydrate Diet and a normal diet. She still had symptoms but avoided letting her symptoms get so bad that she's in serious trouble. Her mother believes that our culture of fast foods and restaurants pushes all the wrong foods. Her goal is to help get her whole family as healthy as can be, but she knows that temptation abounds with foods that are poison to our systems.

We live in a country that offers freedom to make choices, a principal with which I agree. My interest is to provide information so that people can make better informed choices. In the case above, Cara knows she can be medication and symptom free. She is consciously choosing to accept a level of medications and symptoms that she finds tolerable as it fits with her lifestyle choices. I wish her choices had been different and so does her mother, but at least now Cara knows there's something out there that works.

Media Attention

The Specific Carbohydrate Diet occasionally makes the national news. *What is the Specific Carbohydrate Diet?,* an article by Anna Medaris Miller, appeared on the U.S. News and World Report website in 2017.

Miller starts with a story about a 2 ½ year old child being helped by the Specific Carbohydrate Diet. The little girl in infancy had ear infections that were treated with doses of antibiotics. Following the antibiotics, the child's digestive processes didn't work well. Eventually the mom was given advice by a nutritionist to try the Specific Carbohydrate Diet which had an almost immediate favorable effect.

Dr. Sheila Crowe, a clinical professor of medicine at The University of California–San Diego and president-elect of the American Gastroenterological Association, suggested in this article that it's not enough data to give a recommendation to try this diet.

The "lack of data" argument almost always shows when a reporter presents the establishment viewpoint. The Specific

Carbohydrate Diet has been around since 1951. It's likely to never have enough data to suit the mainstream medical community. Dr. Crowe, I suspect, would rather have children and adults take medications with potentially severe side effects over eating a diet that's different. Eating according to the Specific Carbohydrate Diet really has virtually no risk - certainly much less risk than many medications.

Miller also quotes a registered dietitian, Niki Strealy, from Oregon who specializes in digestive health. She suggests that such a diet could lead to "disordered eating behaviors."

How would a person feel about a diet if someone is told that it could lead to disordered eating behaviors? That must be something awful, as it sure sounds bad when in truth it's a very healthy way to eat.

Does it Cost More to Become Healthy?

People I have talked to over the years often have a first impression that a diet such as the Specific Carbohydrate Diet will result in increased grocery costs. The reality is that some costs of foods will go down and some will go up. It's not that simple and straightforward.

Areas where food costs are reduced include the elimination of items such as candy, soda pop, and snack foods. Homemade yogurt is cheaper to make as compared to purchasing it at a store. The drawback is the time in making it which could be considered less convenient.

While each case is different, I would not be surprised if the foods costs associated with the Specific Carbohydrate Diet might actually be about the same or even less. There would naturally be more time and effort required in preparing food. When the opportunity for improved health is taken into account, the long-term convenience factor likely favors a good healthy dietary approach.

Today we find some questionable food items offered but marketed as healthy alternatives. When an item can be projected as more healthy, it often brings with it a premium price to us, the consumer. The mark-up is likely a major reason people think that healthy foods choices cost more.

The bottom line for me is that I've been very well served by eating Gottschall's Specific Carbohydrate Diet and discard the present way of "anything goes" eating. My multitude of health conditions have gone away as a result of this different eating pattern. It hasn't been just bowel disease that has gotten better, but other problems such as hay fever.

Here I'm going to make a quantum leap again. I believe the general population would be significantly healthier, medical bills would be substantially reduced, and longer life spans of good health would occur if a diet like the Specific Carbohydrate Diet was used. This line of thinking will be covered in more detail in subsequent chapters.

Chapter 13

What is Normal?

I eat very differently from people I'm around. People often tell me that they're sorry I'm on such a "restricted" diet. I certainly do eat a narrower range of foods. Most eat anything that tastes good or food that is popular. The limited diet leaves me outside the normal. I don't conform in terms of eating. I am abnormal. I accept that.

When I go to restaurants, the first thing I do is talk to the server. "I'm going to be making some special requests for health reasons," I tell them. I ask for meats to be plain with no sauces, gravies, or seasonings. I ask for plain vegetables. While butter is allowed on the diet, sometimes servers don't know if they use real butter and need to go ask the chef or manager. As a result, I ask for plain. At one restaurant, the manager had no idea what was in their seasoning, which he'd found out had 19 ingredients!

Other approaches have been tried, but this one seems to work best. Sometimes they ask me questions like, "What are you allergic to?" I politely say that it's too involved for me to explain, and can they accommodate my request? I really don't think that I'm allergic to any foods. There's just a lot of foods I'm healthier without. I experience a high rate of success that my meal arrives correct using this approach. If the restaurant makes a mistake, I don't eat it. I can't afford a setback.

I'm heavily involved in community activities. There's always a situation where snacks and refreshments are offered. Sometimes there's not one food I can eat. I don't eat any of it. People sometimes encourage me to eat something, but I respond with a no, thank you.

Over the years, I've kept the nature and extent of my health issues to myself and family. I've definitely not been open about any of this prior to writing this book. I was brought up to keep personal business to one's self. It's like hiding something even though there are clues that I'm sure lead people around me to suspect there's a reason for my eating different foods than most.

On the surface, having Crohn's disease and eating differently makes me abnormal, different, outside the norm. All the lucky ones can eat candy, junk food, beer, and all those processed foods with ingredients that I can't pronounce. Think of all the chocoholics in the world who'd be devastated to have to permanently give it up. Think of all the vast numbers of people who consume soda who would rather be sick than give it up.

People with Crohn's disease want to be "normal." To people like me, that means to be rid of the horrible symptoms. We want to be like everyone else. Most normal people turn to doctors for help for the cure. I'm convinced that my disease is simply a reaction to some foods. Removal of the culprit foods is one way to get better. The mainstream medical community has chosen to go down the path of reducing inflammation or suppressing the immune system to allow people to eat foods that otherwise cause symptoms. There are lots of drugs on the market to help reduce people's reactions to the food they eat. The following contains a couple of examples of how the mainstream medical community approaches people like me for treatment to make us more "normal".

Humira

Let's start with an inflammation reduction drug called Humira (adalimumab). This treatment is advertised heavily on television to convince sick people to go to their doctors and suggest Humira. Humira is used to treat moderate to severe Crohn's disease, ulcerative colitis, rheumatoid arthritis, and skin conditions like hidradenitis suppurativa and plaque psoriasis. Additional disorders this drug is used for include ankylosing spondylitis (AS) and psoriatic arthritis, among others. This medication is one to try after others have failed. The television commercials do include product warnings. From the manufacturer, here is the safety warning:

"You should discuss the potential benefits and risks of HUMIRA with your doctor. HUMIRA is a TNF blocker

medicine that can lower the ability of your immune system to fight infections. You should not start taking HUMIRA if you have any kind of infection unless your doctor says it is okay.

Serious infections have happened in people taking HUMIRA. These serious infections include tuberculosis (TB) and infections caused by viruses, fungi, or bacteria that have spread throughout the body. Some people have died from these infections. Your doctor should test you for TB before starting HUMIRA, and check you closely for signs and symptoms of TB during treatment with HUMIRA. If your doctor feels you are at risk, you may be treated with medicine for TB.

Cancer. For children and adults taking TNF blockers, Including HUMIRA, the chance of getting lymphoma or other cancers may increase. There have been cases of unusual cancers in children, teenagers, and young adults using TNF blockers. Some people have developed a rare type of cancer called heptasyllabic T-cell lymphoma. This type of cancer often results in death. If using TNF blockers including HUMIRA, your chance of getting two types of skin cancer (basal cell and squamous cell) may increase. These types are generally not life-threatening if treated; tell your doctor if you have a bump or open sore that doesn't heal."

As most people don't read the warnings or pay much attention during the television commercials, the potential side effects are not in the forefront of consideration. Also, the product is not a cure. The manufacturer says that it's a medicine "To reduce the signs and symptoms of..." In my mind, do I want to take the risks outlined above for symptom relief? When I was really feeling poorly, I would've likely taken the chance. When a person is desperate, more risk will be tolerated.

The big problem is that Humira is a medicine that negatively impacts the immune system as mentioned on the manufacturer's website. It can reduce the body's ability to deal with infections through a weakening of the immune system.

The immune system is like a shield that protects people from many factors in the environment to stay healthy. A reduction of the immune system inherently leads to a greater risk of cancer and other disorders. The short-term benefit is the reduction of symptoms. One would think that a strong, healthy immune system would be in a person's best interest in terms of good health.

As explained earlier, autoimmune diseases are ones in which the body is thought to react in an abnormal way to factors in the environment. In my case, my body is thought to react abnormally to foods resulting in Crohn's disease and the associated symptoms. The logic is that my own body's immune system is not working correctly and is attacking me. A drug that suppresses the immune system like Humira, when called into action, blocks the activity of something called the Tumor Necrosis Factor (TNF) which results in a lessening of symptoms. This reduction in symptoms is from the anti-inflammatory effect of the drug. In other words, suppress the immune system, get symptom reductions, and take some potentially big risks.

My thinking is that my body's immune system level is working correctly. The symptoms experienced with Crohn's disease is my body telling me to do something different to get relief. Since the symptoms are in my digestive system, the gut, the clue is to look there first. The challenge is to find a way to discover the culprit or culprits.

I previously mentioned that I eliminated dairy products for months and the result was no impact on symptoms. Today, I'm on a diet that doesn't allow lactose-bearing dairy in addition to other food items. The removing one food at a time to find culprits is a weak approach. In the case where many foods being eaten cause the same negative impact, taking them out of the diet one at a time followed by putting them back in often still leaves a lot of culprits in place.

Now that I eat a diet plan that doesn't allow dairy and a lot of other carbohydrates, I do fine. The common denominator is not at the individual food level, but at the *type* of carbohydrate found in the food level.

This obstacle was overcome in my case when a major revamp of my diet happened, then the impact was found in a lot of foods being simultaneously changed. It turned out that there are lots of foods that I can eat and have minimal to no issues. There are also lots of foods that I don't eat as I see a rise in symptoms.

Imuran

Let's look at another medicine that weakens the immune system. Imuran (generic name azathioprine) is used to suppress the body's immune system when there's an organ transplant. This drug is intended to suppress the immune system in cases thought to be autoimmune diseases, while in the case of the previously mentioned, Humira, the suppression of the immune system is a side effect. This abnormal response from the body can be controlled by an immunosuppressant such as Imuran. Some side effects include nausea, upset stomach, vomiting, diarrhea, loss of appetite, hair loss, or skin rash. Here is the product warning information:

"WARNING: Long-term use of azathioprine may infrequently increase your risk of developing certain types of cancer (e.g., skin cancer, lymphoma). This risk is higher in people using azathioprine after an organ transplant and in children/young adults being treated for certain bowel diseases (such as Crohn's disease, ulcerative colitis). You must be closely monitored by your doctor during treatment and regularly afterwards if your doctor stops treatment with this medication.

Azathioprine may also cause serious (rarely fatal) blood disorders (decreased bone marrow function leading to anemia, low number of white blood cells and platelets). It can lower your body's ability to fight an infection.

Keep all medical and laboratory appointments. Tell your doctor immediately if you develop any of the following signs: unusual skin changes, change in the appearance/size of moles, unusual growths/lumps, swollen glands, swollen or painful abdomen, unexplained weight loss, night sweats, unexplained itching, signs of infection (e.g., fever, persistent sore throat), easy bruising/bleeding, or unusual tiredness."

Again, Imuran is not a cure. It's intended to reduce symptoms and brings with it risks. Although the risks may not be high, they do exist. My opinion remains that immunosuppressant and anti-inflammatory drugs, if possible, should be avoided.

My specialist wanted me on Imuran at one point, so I agreed to try it. I remembered the story of one of my support group friends who came to a meeting and told of his experience using an immunosuppressant. He went into remission and was ecstatic, stating he'd never felt better in many years. He continued to come to meetings and report on the big success. We all felt so happy for him. Unfortunately, after about two years, the favorable effect wore off and the drug was no longer useful for him. He reverted back to suffering as before.

My trial with Imuran was much shorter than that of my support group friend. I experienced dizziness after taking the pills, like I'd had too much alcohol to drink. I reported this side effect and was asked to reduce the dosage by 50%. I was a little less dizzy after the change, but it was still a problem. The specialist ended the Imuran trial due to the side effect. I couldn't function while taking it.

Imuran and Humira are simply drugs that treat symptoms and are intended for the patient to be able to eat like everyone else. There is a huge temptation to go this direction as many feel there is no alternative. But there is.

Since only a small percentage of the population has Crohn's disease, that makes me abnormal. All those "lucky" people who are normal can drink beer, eat chocolate, drink soda, and a long list of other goodies. The normal ones don't get symptoms, or so we think. When I eat something I don't tolerate well, within a day or so I get a reaction. Cause and effect are closely tied together in the gut. In normal people, they don't get the short-term feedback that I get. They feel reasonably well and go about their merry way eating whatever appeals to them. They eat candy and snacks and enjoy it all the while possibly long-term problems are developing. The so-called normal person who doesn't have an immediate response to foods that are "not healthy" may not associate their eating habits with the long-term results such as overweight, early onset of heart disease, or other significant disorders.

As I reflect on the long-term results of eating, the "restricted" diet, I've found there has been a very significant side benefit. I've already mentioned earlier that my hay fever symptoms cleared up among others. I theorize that my immune system is no longer reacting to the foods that I eat and is now more able to deal with pollens in the air. When Crohn's disease symptoms heavily weighed me down, I also was sickly in other ways such as colds and flu. My "limited" diet has brought with it no colds, no flu, and no other bugs that go around. Those healthy "normal" people are the ones getting sick and now I'm the "abnormal" one who doesn't get sick.

My body chemistries returned to normal after the diet changes. The doctors could find no reason to prescribe any medications. I just didn't get sick. I felt good all the time.

I think about my high school classmates. I was the sick one all through school and after. Now that we're in our later years, I hear about cases of cancer, heart conditions, strokes, and other serious maladies. I sincerely believe my health challenges went away by eating "abnormally" and have experienced the best health of my life since the change.

Would my ill classmates be willing to make changes like I did, or would they prefer to eat for enjoyment? I suspect the latter as most people who react badly to some foods like I do would ordinarily go to doctors for help, like the majority. My thought now is that I'm far better off having Crohn's disease and eating accordingly to control the symptoms. It's resulted in a higher quality of life and what I feel, a significant increase in longevity for me.

All that I lose in the process is some just foods and other foods that aren't good for my health and well-being. Further, I have no need for medications that treat symptoms that in some cases have potentially serious side effect risks. I don't have a need for even aspirin. I don't experience headaches.

As a person who has successfully made it to retirement, the scenario is quite different with a lot of health issues resolved. There was a journey to get there. That journey was over a very circuitous path that led to a very logical approach when viewed in hindsight. Much of the information is readily available. We just need to connect the dots.

But right now, I'm pretty happy being "abnormally" healthy.

Chapter 14

Restricted and Indulgent

recently was talking to an older couple about their elementary school age grandson who'd been diagnosed with Crohn's disease. The young man had gone through treatment regimens and was not progressing. The mom and dad were faced with a decision for the boy to go on a significant drug treatment that offered a chance of remission, but coupled with some potentially serious side effects. This poor child had experienced bowel resection surgery with about one foot of intestine removed. It's pretty scary for the family to be faced with this significant illness with limited alternatives presented by their doctors. Even more worrisome is that the treatments up to that point had apparently failed.

I told his grandparents that the likelihood of the boy going into remission by using the Specific Carbohydrate Diet was very high. Elaine Gottschall had told me many times that the chance of a favorable result was 95%. It offered an opportunity to return to good health and be medication free. I also advised that complete compliance with the rules of the diet would be required and they would know in less than three weeks if it was going to be effective.

In our discussions about diet and the potential to improve his condition, the word "restrictive" came up. Most people think they can eat anything with minimal or no issues. For example, my own medical specialist told me that he can eat anything with no problem. While he seems to be healthy, he is somewhat overweight.

I mentioned to the grandma and grandpa that the foods I proposed to take out of his diet included (but were not limited to) candy, soda pop, pizza, and similar items. If a young child doesn't eat these things, then they fall into the category of being "different" compared to their peers. Kids want to be part of the group. They want to do things that others do. They don't want to stand apart in those ways. They don't want restrictions.

I followed up and found out later that the grandson ended up on a pretty heavy-duty medication rather than trying the diet. The grandparents wanted to, but the mom was the final decision maker and chose medications over diet. The result in this case is pretty typical of what I've seen over the years.

I personally follow the Specific Carbohydrate Diet 100% exactly. I don't want to suffer the consequences of cheating. I want the benefits that have enabled me to be prescription medication free while not even getting minor health issues. I now have no interest in traditional items such as soda pop, pizza from a nearby pizza store, or candy. I don't drink alcohol or use tobacco. However, other diets do allow alcohol, which we'll discuss in Part 3 of this book.

The Overweight Battle

Almost 69 percent of adults over age twenty are either overweight, obese, or extremely obese.[20] Health issues are known to be higher for those overweight.

The risks associated with overweight people include type 2 diabetes, high blood pressure, heart disease, stroke, cancer, sleep apnea, osteoarthritis, fatty liver disease, kidney disease, and pregnancy problems.[21] So, even if people who eat the typical American diet may not have major problems in the short term, the long term brings with it significant risks for more health issues and a shorter life span.

I look at health similar to the way I looked at safety in the factories that I worked. We were taught that the more safety near misses, the more likely a serious accident would occur. The more likely serious accidents occur, the more likely that a life-threatening accident would result. On the health side, I believe that as people experience increases of minor health issues, the more likely a major health issue will occur. The more major issues occur, the more likely a life-threatening issue will occur.

In my surroundings, I see people as they age starting to experience those minor issues such as colds, hay fever symptoms, or an occasional bout of influenza which they didn't have in their younger years. The frequency of doctor visits rise and more and more prescription medications are used. The message that the body is sending these people is that the immune system is not doing as well as in the past and deterioration of the body is occurring. The protection the body's immune system offers is declining. Eventually, a major disorder such as heart attack, stroke, or cancer is more likely to occur due to a weakened immune system caused in part by aging, but also by lifestyle choices.

There are foods I call indulgent foods. Examples include soda pop, alcohol products, popular candy items, doughnuts, and many more. They're not really on anyone's recommended food lists. They're on the list to consume no more than some in small amounts. If a food is recommended to eat "no more than", I think it would be better not to eat it at all. A person can live quite well without soda, for example.

Now, if a person is stranded on a desert island, that person would eat whatever was available to survive. If soda pop and candy were all there was to eat, then that's what they would eat. If there's more choices, then one would logically go to the healthiest food first and eat the least healthy last. This concept is really important. Our society tends to treat all foods as equally healthy when they're really not.

I contend that most people eat an indulgent diet which in our society is considered normal. On the other hand, I eat what many consider to be a healthy diet 100% of the time without exception with excellent health results, but society makes me a bit of an outcast. Indulgent is normal and restricted is abnormal has been my experience.

Overweight people, when they get to the point where they become concerned about their weight, turn to diets for help. It's dizzying in the number of weight loss diet programs available in the marketplace. It's gotten to the point that diet and overweight are nearly synonymous. When I tell someone I'm on a diet, I get funny looks since I'm now at normal weight for my height.

I know a fellow who struggles with his weight. He eats normally and his weight goes up. He eats foods conducive to weight gain. His diet includes pie, cake, ice cream, and other tasty delights. He appears to really enjoy the foods he eats. In the past, he's tried a commercially available weight loss program under a doctor's supervision. Voila, he lost weight. Then, once the weight goal was achieved, he returned to eating his "normal". It was no surprise that the weight came back. After the weight returned, he went back again to the same weight loss diet and doctor and again got the weight loss he was looking for. Guess what? He returned again to his normal diet and the pounds returned.

For overweight people, there are weight loss pills, weight loss exercise programs, and operations in addition to diet changes. There are many approaches for this market of people that has been steadily growing over the years. Some people unwilling to change their eating patterns resort to gastric bypass surgery. The idea here is that the person feels full sooner and will eat less. Also, some foods will be less tolerated leading the person to want to make diet changes. I think this is a pretty severe approach.

I eat what others call a restricted diet 100% of the time. When I talk to dieticians, they initially don't believe me. They reason that everyone cheats. People often generally do something, but without exception is another matter.

I want to relate an analogy to this concept. When I worked in manufacturing, we tried very hard to supply customers with 100% good quality products to satisfy customers' requirements. This is like my diet all the time. Making 100% good quality product was a very lofty and hard to achieve standard. We worked very hard towards this end. We couldn't *not* follow procedures most of the time and be successful. We had to follow the required procedures all the time. In this line of thinking, I reasoned that I wouldn't be as healthy for the long term if I deviated from the diet plan.

People in their personal lives are not used to following the rules 100% all the time. When people are driving, how many actually follow the speed limits constantly? What percent of drivers really come to a full stop at an intersection before turning right? We know the answer to these two questions are not many.

I believe my short-term health issues are resolved which results in my long-term prospects. I can now be very active. I further believe that my complete turnaround from bad to good health has put me on a path towards improved longevity. While I do have a long history of Crohn's disease and numerous other health issues, by doing what I'm doing, this dreaded disease and my list of other issues are no longer in control.

On one occasion, I had some cake for dessert that was made with ingredients I could eat. I offered my coworker a piece and he asked me if it was healthy. I said yes. Once hearing that, he told me flatly that if it was healthy, he wasn't interested. Some people are like that. What he didn't realize was how tasty my healthy cake was.

If a person wants to live longer than average, be more active than average, and healthier than average, then their approach needs to be different than average. You don't have many options to achieve a long active and healthy life.

People now depend on the healthcare providers to react to health problems once they occur. It would be really good if people were so healthy that their healthcare system dependence was minimized. I suggest that a person can surprisingly improve their overall health and longevity by departing from the norm and eating in a much more healthier way.

In the early to mid 1900's, people smoked tobacco a lot. The incidence rate for men in smoking was always higher than that of women. Today, the percent of the population that smokes is approximately 15%. That's a big change from a majority of people indulging in tobacco use from back then.

Casablanca is a 1942 movie that is among the top films of all time. If you watch the movie, quite a few people smoke tobacco in some of the scenes. Segments in that movie show rooms filled with foggy tobacco smoke. Back in the *Casablanca* era, the person who didn't smoke was different. The analogy is that those who eat those tasty treats and desserts aren't really serving their body well for the long term. Unfortunately, there is no short-term consequence for smoking or poor eating habits. It usually catches up with people over time.

During that time period, those who didn't smoke were different. The people at the time they didn't realize the long-term effects of their tobacco habit such as lung cancer, cardiovascular disease, and a shorter life expectancy. Even with today's knowledge, people still smoke tobacco. Their indulgence might have some serious consequences.

I have a choice in what I eat. I have some idea of the consequences of the "indulgent" way of eating. I'm not going to conform to society's norm. I don't want to be sick and not live as long. I'm thankful to be different, and hope that by reading this book, you understand this philosophy.

Chapter 15

Interacting with Others

O ver the years, I've talked to many people with digestive disorders about the Specific Carbohydrate Diet. I would really like for others to achieve the benefits that I've enjoyed. Now I'd like to share some of the numerous stories based on what I found out from interacting with others.

I received a telephone call from a total stranger one day wanting to talk about how I'd overcome Crohn's disease. While I didn't broadcast my condition a whole lot, occasionally I'd receive referrals from others that did know, and this was one of them.

She expressed a great concern about her health and failure to improve while under a doctor's care. She'd do whatever it would take to get better. We agreed to meet and discuss it. I suggested that we meet at my house. My wife would be there to share her observations of how sick I had been and how I'd improved to the point of needing no medications. The caller was excited and a time and date was set.

Helping this woman seemed not only to be a good thing, but the right thing to do. I was committed to try and help people.

I made a plan of the agenda for the meeting. She would want to tell me her story and I would counter with a short version of my history. Then we would discuss what would be required to go forward and I would also provide her with a copy of Breaking the Vicious Cycle that had all the information she would need. Subsequent to the meeting, I could be called about questions and additional help that would be needed.

She wanted the meeting as soon as possible, so only a few days lapsed until the time of the appointment. I was going to be talking about how to overcome an incurable disease. Isn't that the normal realm of doctors and specialists? I was neither of those. I was an anecdote, a testimonial, certainly not proof. Proof can only be found in official medical studies and clinical trials.

While my case is not part of a scientific study, my health improvement did happen. I am real. I believe that I'm not just a chance happening like winning the lottery. I'm not a fluke.

The day arrived and the woman came with her boyfriend. He was unexpected but welcome as well. We sat and began our discussion.

She talked and talked. She had a story pent up inside that she wanted to share. She covered her suffering, symptoms, and distress. Then she said what sounded like key words: "I would do anything" to get better. I thought that meant she was extremely desperate for relief.

Her detailed story of failed treatments by doctors was all too familiar. As the time passed, it seemed that she was really meeting with me to talk, to express her story. Was she really looking for sympathy, or help? I started to sense it might be the former. The boyfriend said little. I guessed he was there just to provide moral support.

Much of her trials and tribulations I had experienced, although hers were at a lesser level. She had a healthy appearance and carried what one would consider to be a normal body weight. After hearing her lengthy pitch and from my observations, I concluded she was an ill person but hadn't reached a serious point yet.

Eventually the conversation shifted and I was able to tell a brief version of my history confirmed by my wife who patiently participated. Afterwards, I transitioned to talking about diet and its importance. Continuing along that line, I discussed how the mainstream medical community believed that diet has no impact on Crohn's disease. I presented both sides of the story. Our guest already had heard that food or diet was not a factor.

She reiterated her high level of desperation, again contending she was willing to do anything. I believed she was sincere and I took what she said at face value.

I presented *Breaking the Vicious Cycle* to her as a gift and giving her a brief tour to show her how to use it. I pointed out the pages that were key to getting started. I suggested reading it from cover-to-cover before beginning. It would not take long as half the book was text and half recipes.

She would know within three weeks if the diet was going to help. It would take longer than that to get the full benefit, but she could expect a strong signal that she was on the right track. Further, she was told no cheating was allowed. That is tough. In our culture, cheating on diets is the norm not the exception. I further told her that the probability that this diet would help was very high, likely in the 95% range. That's hard for someone new to this concept to comprehend. All she had known up until now was treatments that failed. She was another textbook result of "no known cure".

She accepted the book and told us that she was committed to going forward with this eating regimen. She couldn't wait to get started. She was excited. I was excited for her. I felt that I was living up to my commitment to help others and felt very good about the meeting.

Several months went by and I hadn't heard from her. I was curious but wasn't going to initiate any contact.

One day when I was out doing some shopping, I ran into her. We exchanged greetings after which I asked how she was doing with the diet. She responded with, "I have the book on the shelf and haven't gotten to it yet." It totally deflated me, but I was able to maintain my outward composure.

I realized at that point that she wasn't going to even try. My efforts were in vain. I had failed. I needed to think how to do better in the future.

One of the biggest mistakes I made was giving her the book. It was free to her. Maybe if she'd paid for it, she might've wanted to get a return on her investment. From that day forward, I refused to give items like books for free to help people. I wasn't helping someone who needed to help themselves. I could only provide a road map but couldn't cause them to get out on the diet road and follow it.

Another case came through a friend at work. He and I shared hobbies and interests. We're both ham radio operators and musicians in the community band. We both had daughters in the high school band. We visited and talked frequently.

On one occasion, he mentioned the health issue of his niece, his sister's daughter. She was in her early twenties and struggling with Crohn's disease. I told him my approach would very likely help and could even possibly put her into remission. I shared some of my personal health history and told him that the only help I'd ever gotten was through diet and not through medicines.

My friend didn't know if her version of Crohn's disease was mild, moderate, or severe. He just knew the diagnosis.

He asked how I could get him the information so he could relay it to his sister. I'd order the book and give it to him when it arrived.

As we were waiting for it, he told me of the telephone call with his sister who was very interested. When the book arrived, he insisted on paying for it.

Several weeks went by and I asked him what was happening. He said his sister had read the book and was trying to convince her daughter to try the diet. I appreciated the update and hoped she would try it.

After a few months, I learned his niece wasn't interested in trying it. She instead signed up to be in a program at a major medical center in Chicago in the trial of an experimental drug. My friend and his sister were both disappointed with her decision, but it was her choice.

Several months later, my friend came to me and we sat down to talk. He shared some very bad news with me. His niece had died. The cause of death was complications resulting from the experimental drug she was taking. It was a very sad conversation.

I didn't say much at the time, but my thoughts were strong. Maybe if I'd gotten the information to her sooner it could have made a difference. I had failed again. Over the years, I heard stories like this several times. Very sad and in my view, unnecessary.

In my continuing quest to help people, I found in a nearby city there was a support group for people with digestive problems. I started going as I thought I had learned enough to help people. I really wanted to help sick people get better!

Two very caring ladies organized and headed up the group. They were really into support. When people were in the hospital, they would visit. They published a newsletter to keep people informed.

I met some amazing people. I met a man who had undergone 25 operations in the preceding 25 years. I met a person who worked at a school and had incurred in a year one-third of his employer's (a school system) medical expenses. This was mind boggling. There was the lady who traveled from Indiana to New York for her routine visits to her specialist. I met people who were on total disability who were in better shape than I'd been in my past. It brought me to the realization that I really was a disabled person who, through a combination of fortunate factors, struggled and somehow avoided that fate. I could've given up on working. These were people who were struggling for answers.

I met several people who had so little bowel remaining that they lived on total parenteral nutrition (TPN). That means they're fed nutrition by it being pumped into a vein. The people I met carried a bag with fluid and a battery-operated pump as they went about their normal activities. The "food" was very expensive, thousands of dollars per month. One lady I met had exhausted her $1,000,000 lifetime insurance benefit due to total parenteral nutrition. She petitioned the insurance company for another $1,000,000 and was granted it. Failure for her to have a method to supply her body nutrition meant certain death. She also told me that she felt sick every single day as a result of the way she received nutrition, but she had no choice. There was one member who loved bread. On her way home from grocery shopping, a drive she said took over half an hour, she'd eat a whole loaf of bread in the car. That sounded like something not good for anyone's health!

It was very interesting to hear the members talk about their specialists. They expressed opinions on bedside manner and technical capabilities. Discussions about many local doctors occurred over time - stories of experiences with doctors and changes of doctors and why they changed.

Crohn's Colitis Foundation

After I'd attended support group meetings for a while, representatives from the Indiana Crohn's Colitis Foundation (CCF) state headquarters office came to visit the ladies heading up the local group. They wanted them to have the group associate with the state and national organizations. The CCF has historically worked on finding cures by raising funds and distributing the funds to help in research.

The leaders of the local group quickly found out the CCF's interest in the local group was mostly of a fundraising nature. The foundation itself states it's a "non-profit, volunteer-driven organization dedicated to finding the cures for Crohn's disease and ulcerative colitis"[22] The local leaders were less interested in finding cures and more interested in helping people deal with the problems they were experienced.

The matter of the CCF was brought to the local group for discussion who decided not to affiliate with CCF, but agreed to hold one annual fundraising event to raise money for them.

I attended many support group meetings but met with little if any success in getting interest in my suggestion that changing foods can help. I wasn't particularly interested in the CCF and helping them to find the cure as I was already much improved without any new "cure" being needed.

The CCF has commented on the Specific Carbohydrate Diet. The CCF points out that the Specific Carbohydrate Diet is "supported only by testimonials, not by systematic studies."[23]

Further, the CCF website has a link to a paper (from their Specific Carbohydrate Diet (SCD) page) to a *Journal of Pediatric Gastroenterology & Nutrition* entry. This article suggests that "Many diet therapies for Crohn's disease are known to be effective."[24] The conclusion of this paper states that "The apparent effectiveness of the Specific Carbohydrate Diet in Crohn's Disease warrants more study."[25]

The CCF references a second paper also accessed by a link from their Specific Carbohydrate Diet page that states "Although the exact time of symptom resolution could not be determined through chart review, all symptoms were notably resolved at a routine clinic visit 3 months after initiating the diet."[26] From the conclusion section of the paper, it's suggested that the SCD and other low complex carbohydrate diets may be useful for Crohn's disease.

The CCF is a large organization that according to its 2014 annual report had total contributions, grants, and other income and support totaling $77,269,154. Founded in 1967, CCF's stated mission is "To cure Crohn's disease and ulcerative colitis, and to improve the quality of life of children and adults affected by these diseases." After 50 years of effort, they are still looking to find the cure. When I think about foundations like this, the polio case comes to mind.

The National Foundation for Infantile Paralysis was the organization that worked towards the cure for polio. Once polio was eradicated, there was no longer a need for the national fundraising organization. The organization continues to exist today with a name change and a new mission. Now called the March of Dimes, it works on birth defects. Should the cure for inflammatory bowel disease come along, the CCF could follow the pattern set by the current March of Dimes as long as a suitable new cause can be found or otherwise go out of business.

If cures are found, the foundations that support those cures will either go out of business or find a new cause as the polio folks did. Employees in such organizations surely want to stay employed, so there's an advantage to not finding a cure.

CCF Proposal

I'd like to propose a small study to CCF This organization spends millions of dollars each year on research and studies related to bowel disease.

There are people with bowel disease with varying levels of symptoms. In my case, once the disease set in, there wasn't even one day free of symptoms. My symptoms were terrible each and every day. I'm presuming there are lots of folks around the country in the same condition.

My suggestion is for CCF researchers to hire one person and pay that person a significant wage. The person should have severe symptoms that occur each and every day. That person should be isolated at a research facility and plan on the activity taking around three months.

The first few weeks of the study would be to provide the person under study with food as similar as possible to what they were eating before the study. The researchers should carefully document how the gut reacts, as in symptoms.

After several weeks of documentation and verification, this person should be put on the Specific Carbohydrate Diet. Conditions need to be controlled throughout so the person has no access to food other than what the researchers provide. The results would be documented on a daily basis for the next few weeks.

While this is a simplified version of what would be needed, it's certainly not a study that would require millions and millions of dollars. The key would be finding the right person who always has symptoms. Since the disease is considered by experts to be incurable and not caused by food, it should lead to a good test.

In the field of statistics, large studies are needed to detect small changes, while small studies are needed to detect large changes. My suggestion of studying one sick person is based on the idea that I believe a large favorable change will occur. I think it would surprise many regarding the results that could be achieved by studying one subject.

Once the first study is done, there's no doubt more would be done to verify. The biggest challenge is to get that first study accomplished.

Chapter 16

Answers Based on My Experiences

As a person who's had many health issues in life, I've found that by changing my diet, my health improved dramatically. I never in this world would have believed that such a huge change was possible. I developed a theory as to how this works.

By means of an analogy, let's say a person is out in the sun a lot and gets sunburned. Their skin becomes irritated and painful. In fact, the person likes being out in the sun, which continues to worsen the skin discomfort. The person eventually starts to get ill. Their health goes into decline. Figure 17-1 shows a graphical depiction of the impact of sunburn.

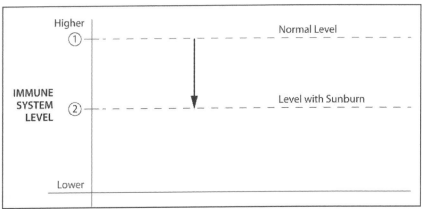

Figure 17-1. Immune system impact from sun exposure.

The immune system impacted goes from Level 1 to Level 2, and the affected person becomes more susceptible to other symptoms and conditions. Eventually, this hypothetical person goes to the doctor and describes the skin condition and the health symptoms.

The person tells the doctor a treatment, a cure is desired. The doctor looks at the patient and says the skin and health issues are due to sun exposure. For the short term, there are some medications that will help treat the skin. The doctor continues by saying that the sunburn will decrease with less sun exposure. This seems pretty obvious. Now let's take a look at a case which is typical for those with Crohn's disease or any bowel disease.

A person eats food and lots of digestive symptoms develop. The digestive system becomes irritated. The person not only needs food to survive but eats many foods they enjoy. The symptoms continue and worsen over a long period of time. The person's overall health is in decline. Finally, the person goes to the doctor and describes the digestive and health symptoms. Now in this case, the doctor tells the patient that this is Crohn's disease for which there is no known cause or cure. For the short and long term, there are medications and operations that will help the current situation. The doctor tells the patient that foods eaten are not the problem. The patient lives a life with medications and operations with the associated high medical bills and much discomfort.

Now let's do another version of the same story. A person eats food and gets lots of digestive symptoms. The digestive system becomes irritated and pain is incurred. The person not only needs food to survive but eats many foods they enjoy. The symptoms continue to worsen over a long period of time. The person's overall health is in decline. Finally, the person goes to the doctor and describes the digestive and health symptoms. This doctor tells the patient that this is Crohn's disease and the body is reacting to the foods eaten. The doctor advises the patient to eat according to the Specific Carbohydrate Diet and to do so 100% of the time for two to three weeks to verify it will be effective.

The patient returns to the doctor three weeks later and reports that the symptoms have greatly improved. The doctor is pleased with the patient's improvement. The doctor advises the patient that the load on the immune system is reduced (see Figure 17-2) and the overall sense of well-being should improve. The patient is eating selected fruits, vegetables, nuts, and meats along with some lactose-free dairy. The patient feels healthier than they have in years and is very happy with the improvements. The patient is surprised that no medications are needed, and as a result, medical bills are very low.

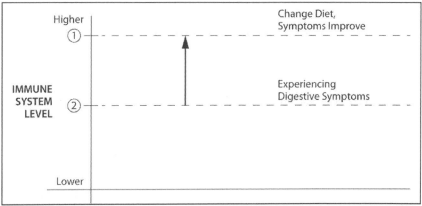

Figure 17-2. Eating a diet that reduces digestive symptoms results in the immune system being favorably impacted.

The sunlight causing sunburn in the first story is analogous to the foods eaten causing digestive tract symptoms in the 2nd and 3rd versions of the story. In the real world, no one would go to the doctor for a cure for irritated skin caused by continued exposure to the sun. That is exactly what people do for their long-term digestive distresses, reactions to the foods eaten. Most people who are diagnosed with Crohn's disease and ulcerative colitis end up like the second version of the story, lives filled with medications, operations, high medical costs, and low quality of life.

That addresses the case of a person with obvious digestive distress. Earlier, I covered the years when I had many symptoms that didn't include my digestive system. When I changed the diet, those symptoms disappeared. This brings me to a very important point. The food that we eat can negatively impact our body's immune system making us susceptible to symptoms such as hay fever. We don't realize the root cause and the hay fever is treated.

The further and further we get away from eating the optimal mix of foods to satisfy nutritional needs, the more likely we are to have minor and major health issues. It's most certainly in our best interest as a society to figure out what this "optimal" food eating plan is. Moving towards an optimal diet, we can expect it to raise the level of the immune system. This outcome is shown in figure 17-3 and results simultaneously in maximizing our good health.

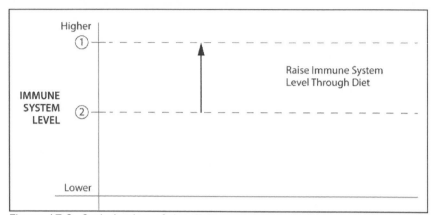

Figure 17-3. Optimization of the diet can take load off the immune system leaving valuable immune system resources available to deal with other issues.

I've learned a lot over the years from dealing with my health as well as my interaction with the healthcare system. Much of it has surprised me given where I am now and how I arrived there. Both successes and failures have been experienced from within the system while there have been some very favorable results achieved from the fringes of the mainstream medical world.

I have so clearly found that food eaten is far more important to my well-being than I could have imagined, and I believe it extends to other people as well. I'm convinced that foods we ingest are far more important than most realize. In thinking about my experience, I wonder what I could've done earlier to avoid being so sick.

Had I eaten the Specific Carbohydrate Diet all my life, much if not all of my illnesses might've been avoided. I might not have had pneumonia three times. I might have been free of airborne allergies. I might never have experienced the symptoms of ankylosing spondylitis (AS). I might never have experienced the symptoms of Crohn's disease. I might not have incurred a significant skin condition. Many medical expenses such as doctor bills, prescriptions, and operations may not have been needed. My family had no way of knowing what diet I needed and as I grew into adulthood, I didn't realize the ties my symptoms had to diet. I only changed my food selection in reaction to my symptoms and disease; otherwise, I wouldn't have changed my foods.

Our healthcare system today works the same way. Once symptoms show up, there is a reaction in the form of a treatment. People are presumed healthy unless symptoms or test results point to the contrary. This is not a good presumption.

Planning Ahead

Food choices can be deliberately planned to create good health, not only just for me, but for everyone. The diet would need to be determined before there were symptoms and illnesses. This thinking led me to the possibility that good health and longevity could both be improved while significantly reducing healthcare costs.

The conclusion I've drawn is that good health starts with the gut. We need to eat foods that work well with our digestive tracts. Foods that commonly irritate the gut are thought to only impact a small part of the population. That's wrong. Some foods cause us problems even without resulting symptoms. The gut is acting like a screening mechanism to warn or tell us not to eat some foods. Unfortunately, the reactions to foods eaten varies a lot among people.

Only a small part of the population has Crohn's disease, around a 0.5% rate. My DNA testing indicates that I'm 8 times more likely than the general population to have Crohn's disease. Based on that test results, it indicates a 4% chance of contracting the disease. My propensity is to have bowel disease and bowel disease symptoms. Even with significant symptoms, most want to continue to eat problem foods, so they turn to medications and operations to keep going. Little do they realize that the people viewed as not having gut issues are also being impacted by the same foods.

We think of gut issues as either being there or not being there. What I think is really happening is that some have the gut issues from the foods, but others are also being impacted by the same foods and either have no symptoms or have symptoms not associated with gut issues.

There really is no way to predict most illnesses people will incur with great accuracy in terms of what and when. The common denominator is that many people eat foods implicated with digestive issues and according to my thinking, lowers the effectiveness of the immune system. As we age, this impact grows as do minor and major health issues. As the immune system becomes less effective, health and longevity are directly impacted.

There's a tune Cole Porter wrote many years ago called *Anything Goes*. It's a fun and bouncy piece of music which goes together with the title. That's how we think of food. Whatever we like, enjoy, meets a cost objective, or is prepared in a timely fashion that works for many. Our society's "anything goes" diet practices are so varied that direct correlations and understanding are hard to detect and understand.

Now that I have my immune system operating at a higher level through diet as referenced in Figure 17-3, I've become less susceptible to many health conditions. As a person raises the level of their immune system through diet, their overall health and healthcare costs will go down resulting in the opportunity for new levels of longevity and good health.

One concept that will be tough for the reader to overcome is the one which says action should be taken in a reaction mode. Certainly, we need to react to illness and injury, but it would be much better to plan ahead and either not have or minimize future health distresses.

In business situations, managers try to be proactive to minimize risks, and try to anticipate and prevent problems from occurring in the first place. Taking the proactive idea to health suggests we assume that all people have the potential to be sick and measures should be taken in advance so that illnesses are minimized or never occur.

Starting with the premise that all people are either going to be sick or are sick, there could be a diet plan in place for each person or a general diet plan that forms the basis or foundation for eating. By consuming this yet-to-be-determined food plan, the human body will be functioning well and the body's own immune system will be expected to fend off many illness threats.

The principal emphasized in my experience with exposure at the office to sulfur dioxide, I found that people don't all react to the same issue the same way. Some have no symptoms while others have symptoms at various levels. Exposure to a poisonous gas over time is bad for everyone, yet some experienced no ill effects. For those with no symptoms, the exposure was still just as bad.

Many people can eat foods their body seems to tolerate well, but actually, the body is not functioning as well, resulting in lower immune system protections. As shown in Figure 17-4, while symptom free, a person's immune system at Level 2 is unknowingly impacted. This yields the potential of more illness and shorter lifespan in the long haul. For example, when hay fever season rolls around, some of the Level 2 folks move to Level 3 and start to exhibit symptoms. Unfortunately, these people don't realize that their diet coupled with the pollens in the air are the root cause.

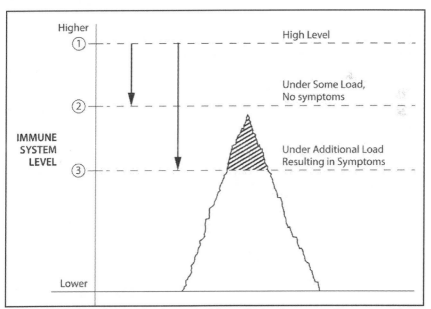

Figure 17-4. People can be impacted by a factor in a negative way with no resulting symptoms.

A symptom-free person can function internally at a lower, less efficient level, rendering them more susceptible to illness and disease over time. And not realizing their immune system is being pulled down to a lower level of effectiveness.

Let's consider how two people can be exposed to the same issues and have different results as illustrated in Figure 17-5. Person A and Person B in Figure 17-5 are different, as we all are. We each have a different DNA, a unique lifestyle and environment that comes from the freedoms we have to make choices within reasonable boundaries.

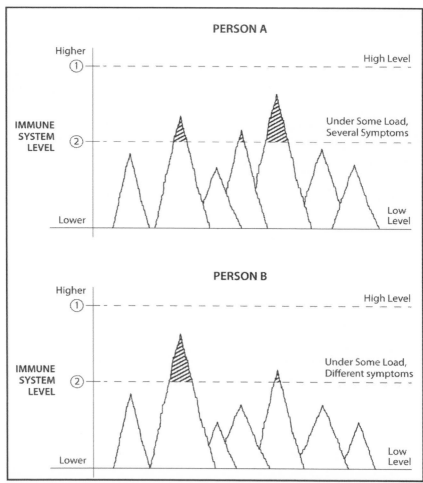

Figure 17-5. Person A & Person B have different susceptibilities. Both people can be impacted differently by being exposed to the same negative factors.

The analogy made in Figure 17-5 is the mountain ranges shown on the charts are like DNA. The two-example people have two different DNA's (or mountain ranges). When these two people experience something that causes their immune system to go from Level 1 to Level 2, they don't experience the same results in the same way. Their peaks have different heights with each peak being a different symptom or response.

The food people ingest is a controllable factor. People can change the diet and achieve a higher level of health which will result in a more robust immune system to deal with daily issues. Controllable factors are really the lifestyle choices we make.

Let's take alcohol consumption as an example. In the short term, people who consume alcoholic beverages enjoy the experience. Seemingly healthy, they may experience the "buzz" and find that a desirable result. That buzz is actually a signal that something is wrong. People just don't recognize it as such. They, in many cases, are getting what they want.

The long term brings with it the opportunity for alcohol-related illnesses and potentially a shorter lifespan from diseases such as cirrhosis of the liver, cancer, and cardiovascular disease. Alcoholism can lead to life spans reduced by 5 to 10 years. Alcohol is a consumable item that is on the list of items that adversely affect the body and the immune system. This idea extends to other foods that people eat, but usually not as dramatically.

There are foods that the body can effectively digest that gives the various organs of the body the "food" needed for good health and functioning. There are also foods considered edible that humans don't process or digest well. They also don't provide the nutrients the body needs. Another way to say this is that all foods are not equally edible.

Also, for the body to get the optimal nutrition, a combination of foods is needed to satisfy the "chemistry" needs of the various bodily processes.

The idea of what constitutes a healthy diet is very controversial with many viewpoints. The media batters us with bits and pieces daily. Most people just throw up their hands and eat what they like and enjoy. This is consistent with what others eat.

The absence of having a direct measure of the state of the body's immune system leaves us with no way to know the status of our immune system. We do however have indirect measures.

People who have lots of lower level illnesses such as hay fever, influenza, headaches, colds, and similar disorders are really receiving a message from their body that their own immune system is under sufficient load from controllable and uncontrollable factors that it cannot maintain symptom-free health.

The Hardest Change of All

The story about the person with sunburn was discussed followed by a couple of versions of the same story featuring a person with bowel disease. If a person can turn off and turn on a symptom such as sunburn or digestive distress, then a root cause is known. This is important in terms of the concept of autoimmune diseases.

Crohn's disease, celiac disease, Ulcerative Colitis, and other digestive disorders are thought to be a result of the body's own immune system going haywire and attacking the body in the digestive tract. If food is really the root cause, this is likely not the case. The body likely is in fact functioning correctly and sending a message that something in the diet is causing issues.

If these bowel disorders are not autoimmune diseases, what are they? They wouldn't even be diseases. They would be like the relationship between the sun (food) and sunburn (bowel irritation).

The confusing factor in this is that many people don't exhibit bowel symptoms when eating suspect foods. The key here is that on the surface, people appear to be unaffected when, in fact, they are affected.

All of my life prior to making diet changes I suffered from a variety of conditions. Little did I realize those symptoms were caused by what I was eating. The foods were using part of my immune system to the point it could no longer keep me symptom free. I had no way of knowing the connection of my diet to these symptoms until the dietary changes caused them to clear up over time.

If a person wants to raise the effectiveness of their immune system, become healthier, lower medical costs, and live longer, controllable factors such as diet must be modified. The problem is how to measure the results of changes, but an even bigger challenge is how to get people to change.

What we're looking for is an approach that enables the digestive system to function efficiently and effectively while simultaneously reducing and eliminating colds, hay fever, influenza, and other lower level ailments. The big picture we're looking for is a lifestyle that positions a person to minimize the potential to have major serious and life-threatening conditions like heart disease, stroke, and cancer.

Chapter 17

"Normal" People Get Healthier

I have friends who as a couple wanted to lose weight. While they had some health issues, none would be considered major. These people didn't have bowel disease, so ordinarily, they would have no reason to consider a diet intended to improve gut issues. I told the husband that he and his wife could lose weight by excluding some foods while having no quantity restrictions. Eating a variety of fruits, vegetables, meats, nuts, and other foods conformed to the diet I use. The look he gave me at the time was really more than skeptical, but he was polite.

The rules they needed to follow would lead him and his wife to the desired result. I told him that their overall health and feeling of well-being would likely improve. He continued to give me funny looks during our discussion, but he didn't totally dismiss me.

I gave him some guidelines for the Specific Carbohydrate Diet. More funny looks. We talked on several occasions and he gradually absorbed what I said to the point that he and his wife made changes.

My friends did not get 100% over to the carbohydrate diet but they did make some major moves toward it.

Here is their story from husband Carl's point of view:

"Diane and I are 51 years old. We were very active in high school playing tennis and track. I went on to play tennis in college. We ate typical farmer-type meals (vitamin D whole milk, bacon, eggs and mashed potatoes) until about age 35 when our metabolisms seemingly overnight shut down.

We didn't go out to eat as often as our friends did. Diane has had severe allergies and I always seem to get strep throat twice a year pretty bad. We also got the flu each year like everyone else.

At age 35, I decided to go on a big exercise kick and trained for a triathlon. I completed two over the next 4 years. I was in great physical shape and this helped Diane also do her own aerobics program. We didn't lose any weight but did feel better.

Then at 40, we really gained more weight with no change in habits. Increased exercise didn't make any difference. We then began a series of yo-yo dieting. We first tried the low-calorie diets such as Weight Watchers and Nutrisystem, which worked for a while, but didn't support our active lifestyle very well, and we still had an abundance of illness from flu, common cold, and Diane's allergies were creating issues with bronchitis.

We then moved to low carb diets such as Atkins and South Beach which we liked better. Our energy level was higher and we got better sleep. I cannot recall why we stopped following these diets; perhaps out of a lack of discipline or not able to truly drop enough weight past a certain point or goal. Either way, no changes in health other than Diane was beginning to have more seasonal asthma issues, and I had very high cholesterol and blood pressure. My doctor advised going on medication.

By age 47, we decided to take a different look at things after meeting with John Chalmers who discussed a very natural type of diet. We began to read about what he was speaking about and came across a book called The Daniel Plan which offered both a spiritual guide as well as a cookbook on eating healthy. This combination of what John was telling us allowed us to reach our weight goals while at the same time, getting healthier.

My blood pressure and cholesterol fell back to an athlete's range and my doctor stopped pushing medication. Diane hasn't had a cold or flu or any asthma issues since. The biggest struggle is just putting in the time to prepare quality meals."

Here is their story from wife Diane's point of view:

"Biggest Positive:
My biggest positive take-away has been health. My weight continues to fluctuate, but my health does not. Since getting

serious about what we put into our bodies, we simply don't get sick anymore. I used to get at least one sinus infection per year, which always would turn into one nasty bout of bronchitis and ultimately asthmatic bronchitis. I then had to go on steroids and inhalers after the antibiotics failed. This was an annual winter cycle with me, and one that I thought I would go through for the rest of my life. I could never sing Christmas songs at church because I always seemed to have a sinus infection during the holiday season. I also had regular headaches and migraines.

These things have entirely disappeared for the last 3 years. I attribute this solely to diet. And full disclosure: I have been inconsistent with the eating program. I function very well on it for 6-12 weeks, then regress, and repeat the cycle. But even with my lack of consistency, the health benefits have amazed me.

Biggest Negative:

My biggest negative with your food program was my lack of knowledge and lack of knowing how to find adequate resources. I have had to entirely relearn to cook. This involves a lot of "unlearning" as I had to throw away everything in my recipe box and start over. I found that I need a lot of information and specifics in order to plan ahead, and to have on-hand what we need in anticipation. For this reason only, I've defaulted to the Daniel Plan recipes and Paleo resources because they were easily accessible and seemed to follow most of the basic principles.

Another negative has been my immediate family. We have tried very hard to never be judgmental of anyone else's food choices; however, my mom especially has struggled. She loves to invite us over for meals, and we just won't eat a lot of what she makes. One of her favorite things to make for everyone is homemade bread. She continues to act as if we've hurt her feelings every time we refuse to eat bread. We have taken our own food, invited her to our house (and they always LOVE what we prepare), but changing our eating program has also impacted others in our family. This will not cause us to make any changes but has been an issue sometimes for me. To make this broader, I would say that so much of our lives now combines meals and social elements, and I haven't quite figured out how to combine them both in all cases.

Carl and I have a very busy lifestyle by choice, which means that the other negative has been the amount of time we need to dedicate to this relearning process, planning, grocery shopping, and cooking. Carl has been an amazing partner in the kitchen as he now helps. That has made all the difference in the world. If I were to be relearning this alone, I would have had even more slips.

As our community continues to promote farm to table and local food choices, it becomes easier to learn about the benefits of a clean, healthy diet. (Today for lunch, we had chicken/cauliflower soup (buffalo chicken soup) loaded with veggies and deviled eggs made with avocado and lemon juice instead of mayonnaise and mustard. They were wonderful, but I certainly had to have a recipe to follow the first time.)

Carl and I talked about this. Both of our favorite recipes continue to be those that "fool" our heads into thinking we haven't given up anything with this new program. Our logical mind knows that to be healthy, we need to make certain choices. But the emotional side thinks that we still need to eat the foods (comfort foods) that we grew up on. So our favorites are the recipes that allow us to continue to eat all of our favorites.

Pizza was a tough one for us to give up. By learning how to use cauliflower to make a pizza crust, and then adding Italian spices, we now feel like we eat pizza as often as we want. We realized that the crust had no flavor anyway; the flavor simply came from the tomatoes and spices. Cauliflower is our new favorite food. Riced cauliflower in stir fry recipes, the above pizza crust, mashed cauliflower, and roasted cauliflower.

Almond and coconut flour were another great discovery with this program.

I had to align my expectations with the new ingredients. Not everything would taste the same as what I was used to, but once I had eaten clean for a few weeks, my palate would seem to reset itself so healthy and natural foods ended up tasting better than the processed foods. This didn't happen overnight *though and we found it was important to give ourselves a little time to adjust.*

One of my favorite things about your program is that you don't count calories or weigh your foods. If you eat the "right" foods, you don't have to limit yourself beyond normal reasonableness."

The interesting result for this couple was the weight loss combined with the relief from symptoms such as airborne allergies and asthma, as well as the husband's drop from his high cholesterol level. They didn't have to resort to starving themselves for weight loss. Their big issue was eating in conformance to the diet rules. When they departed from their special diet, they suffered the consequences as the symptoms would return and weight would be gained. In other words, they could turn their symptoms off and on depending on the foods eaten. They do have some control.

This couple was not experiencing bowel disease or gut issues of any kind. Other than being overweight, they seemingly had no disorders associated with foods. By eating a diet that was more in tune with gut issues, this couple was able to make significant improvements in non-gut issues. This is significant. I don't have the resources to prove this on a scientific basis, but on an anecdotal basis, this story confirms my thinking that changes in the diet can lead to surprising results.

Another way to verify that food was a culprit became apparent when they strayed from the diet plan. The symptoms they'd experienced returned not immediately, but gradually.

I also asked a fellow named Bart to share his story which follows:

"I have been 20 to 25 pounds overweight. I also have a history of sinus infections over the last 20 years. When I have sinus infections, I'm sick in bed for 1 to 2 weeks at a time. I have a skin condition that concerns me a great deal as it is pre-cancerous in nature. Additionally, I was tested years ago and was found to have nonalcoholic fatty liver (NAFL). This can lead to liver failure if it gets bad enough. I try to avoid things that irritate it.

In the past, I've heard favorable comments about low carb diets and have been dabbling in low carb diets for a couple of decades. I continued to eat grains and sugars but less of them.

When I heard about the Specific Carbohydrate Diet, my impression was that it was more focused as it takes into account the digestibility, not just the carb count. I never thought of digestibility before to help good health.

Now that I have experienced eating according to the Specific Carbohydrate Diet, it does make me feel better in many ways. Now that I am older, the impact seems to be getting greater. My digestion is better and less acidic.

My weight is reduced as long as I stay on the diet plan. When I eat more complex carbohydrates, I gain weight. My blood pressure historically has been borderline high. My weight and blood pressure seem to go up and down together correlating with what is eaten.

My sinus health is noticeably better now too. The effect is almost immediate. I can switch my sinus off and on just by my food choices.

When I eat complex carbohydrates, my pre-cancerous skin lesions flare up resulting in painful red broken places in the skin. This red scaly lesion is a concern and is the result of too many years of sun exposure. When complex carbohydrates are avoided, my skin is healthier and less prone to developing those little sores.

The lure of sweets is very hard to resist. I guess that I have a sweet tooth. My family has a history of diabetes, so you would think that I would know better. When I do eat something with complex carbohydrates, I feel like I have more acid stomach and more gas as well. This was normal for years for me.

I make the homemade yogurt. I bought an inexpensive yogurt maker and ferment the yogurt for over 24 hours rather than the 4.5 hours given in the instructions. I like yogurt and it is cheaper for me to make than to buy at the store. I believe that eating this yogurt is good for me and I really enjoy it as does my wife.

Omitting the complex carbohydrates from the diet I believe will not only help the people with digestive diseases but can help the general population as it has helped me. This has been my experience for some time now, even though I stray from the diet from time-to-time."

It gives me great joy to pass on these stories to you. The Specific Carbohydrate Diet will not only help people with digestive diseases but can help the general population as demonstrated by the stories my friends have shared. Good health for anyone is dependent on the body's immune system functioning at a high level. Diets like the Specific Carbohydrate Diet appear to do this.

While there is no direct measure of the immune system, there are numerous indirect indicators. Many tend to discount getting colds, influenza, hay fever, and the like as minor, but they really are not. These so-called "minor" issues are all significant.

Through the gut, my thinking is that there is a significant pathway to improving health and longevity, and that pathway can generally be applied to everyone. In Part 3 of this book, we'll look at the pros and cons of some major diets you might recognize by name.

Part Three

Chapter 18

The Paleo Diet

In my quest to get healthier, I went through three versions of what I eat. The rotation diet plan helped a lot which was helped even more by the Specific Carbohydrate Diet. The Paleo Diet is almost a subset of the diet I now eat. As a result, I think it likely would be very helpful for good health and improve longevity as well.

To provide some history, Paleo is the shortened name for Paleolithic, humans who lived between two and three million years ago. The thought is that this would be the best foods that the human body is best adapted to eat. This idea was popularized by Loren Cordain, PhD in his book, *The Paleo Diet* (later revised in 2011 and released as *The Paleo Diet Revised Edition*).

In reading various websites regarding the Paleo Diet, you might find variations in the diet and possibly not the diet itself. I've read websites that say potatoes are Paleo and others say they're not. Obviously, both are not correct. It's always good to go to a reliable source for information which in this case is the writings of Loren Cordain himself. In the case of white and sweet potatoes, neither are allowed.

This diet is very similar to the Specific Carbohydrate Diet in that sugar, high fructose corn syrup, and foods containing grains are not allowed. However, the Paleo Diet goes even further by making dairy off limits.

Alcohol is allowed on an occasional basis including wine, beer, and other adult beverages. My interpretation of this is that Cordain has recognized some would be unwilling to give up alcohol so he allows it in small amounts. By allowing some alcohol, the number of potential followers of his diet increases. In contrast, the Specific Carbohydrate Diet only allows small amounts of non-grain-based alcohol products such as dry wine.

Dairy is not recommended for the Paleo Diet. The Specific Carbohydrate Diet does allow lactose-free dairy such as homemade yogurt fermented for 24 to 34 hours and fermented brick cheeses. Overall, the Paleo Diet is generally narrower in scope compared to what is allowed on the Specific Carbohydrate Diet.

Now let's cut to the chase and look at some of the Paleo Diet claims. Near and dear to my heart is Crohn's disease. Loren Cordain's book contains the success story of a woman who claims to be 100% symptom free after going on the diet.[27] Cordain puts the blame on Crohn's disease and a laundry list of other digestive disorders onto the American diet with its "overload of refined grains, sugars, dairy, and processed foods."[28]

In a chapter titled Food as Medicine, it covers a vast array of illnesses that he believes originated with poor diet. He claims that "The Paleo Diet is good medicine!"[29] Cordain often takes the position that eating the Paleo Diet will result in a person being much less likely to get heart disease, stroke, or cancer as well as many more disorders.

These claims are rather remarkable. Elaine Gottschall focused mostly on digestive disorders and autism for the Specific Carbohydrate Diet. Cordain takes the claims a lot farther, to the point that he covers most any illness. His list of health issues he believes the Paleo Diet may prevent is so extensive it's too long to include here.

Sounds awfully good, but this presents two problems for me. First, which of the two diets is better for my Crohn's disease? Another way to state this is, do I want to give up my homemade yogurt? Second, are these claims really true? I'm not planning to switch to the Paleo Diet, sticking with the "If it ain't broke don't fix it" argument. Having said that, I have no way of knowing whether it's less effective, equal, or more effective on bowel diseases. I look at the recipes in Cordain's book and many of them are very compatible with what I've been eating. It does seem possible to me that it might be better than the food plan I currently follow, but I do believe if there is a difference, it's small.

Cordain's claims are highly likely accurate, based on my personal experience with a similar diet and with the concepts presented earlier in this book. While I think that it's a very good diet, studies would need to be done to prove it one way or another.

Once the conversation goes to needing scientific studies, we end up at a road block. The studies will never get done. We as individuals can make changes on our own that feature virtually no risk, but the opportunity for improvement is huge. Today's *anything goes* diet that most eat leaves us with known incidence rates of heart disease, cancer, stroke, and bowel disease along with many more. It will take a different approach to get a different result.

Chapter 19

The Lutz and Atkins Diets

I f we were to choose to eat in prevention mode, we would eat foods that we believe would lead to maximum good health and longevity. In the prevention way of thinking, we'd be constantly working towards keeping major issues such as heart disease, stroke, and cancer from ever happening. The problem we're faced with is the selection of a diet that when followed, minimizes health issues.

Earlier in this book, we covered the Specific Carbohydrate Diet and its associated gluten-free feature. This diet can resolve many health issues by addressing issues associated with the body's first line of defense in protecting good health, the gut. The gut to some extent screens out foods that the body doesn't want, but unfortunately, accepts some that are unhealthy as well. Following that same line of thought, the Paleo Diet is similar in nature and there are claims of its favorable impact on health being extensive.

There are so many diets out there, there's enough information available for many volumes. Most people think of diets and dieting as associations to weight loss or reactions to health issues. With more than half of the United States population overweight or obese, there are many diet offerings which address overweight issues. However, the choice of foods to be eaten should really go far beyond weight control.

A person who wants to never have a heart attack could take the approach of eating a heart healthy diet as a preventive measure. A person who doesn't want to have diabetes could eat a diet recommended for that purpose. A person who wants to avoid celiac and other bowel diseases could eat a diet used for people with those conditions. However, it's not reasonable to eat many different diets all at once which poses a real dilemma.

I believe the Lutz and Atkins diets can help us to have further insight into diet optimization. These two diets have similarities with each other and also are somewhat related to the Specific Carbohydrate Diet and Paleo Diet.

The Lutz Diet, developed by Dr. Wolfgang Lutz, involved over 40 years of research and over 10,000 patients. Dr. Lutz, a native of Austria, developed his low carbohydrate diet to address issues such as diabetes, heart disease, gastrointestinal disorders, weight control, cancer, anemia, and hypertension. His approach to finding solutions appears to be similar to that of Dr. Sydney Haas, whose research of pediatric celiac disease led to the development of the Specific Carbohydrate Diet with Elaine Gottschall.

The results of the Lutz work are summarized in his book, *Life Without Bread: How a Low-Carbohydrate Diet Can Save Your Life* and is coauthored by Christian Allan, Ph.D. The book was originally published in Europe in 1967, about 16 years following Dr. Haas publishing his book.

The Lutz Diet is simple and, in spite of the book title, does allow bread. The diet is described as follows:

"Restrict all carbohydrates to 72 utilizable grams per day. Eat as much of any other foods as you wish."[30]

To clarify this for the reader, 72 grams is 2.54 ounces or a little over 1/8 pound. Given the quantity of food eaten a day, it's not very much. To put this in perspective, the authors of *Life Without Bread* indicate 1 slice of bread contains approximately 12 grams of carbohydrates which he calls a BU (bread unit).[31] So bread is allowed on the diet, but the total quantity of carbohydrates of all types is limited.

To put the 72-gram carbohydrate limit into perspective, some food examples are covered. The United States Department of Agriculture (USDA) has a website which gives access to the USDA Branded Foods Data Base.[32] Let's look at some foods from this database to gain perspective on the amounts of carbohydrate in a serving of various foods.

Cola soda, 20 oz.	65 grams
Instant oatmeal, 41gram packet	27.47 grams
Orange juice, 12 oz.	39.01 grams
100% whole wheat, whole	

grain bread, 1 slice	16 grams
2% reduced fat milk, 1-cup	13.01 grams
Candy bar, 2.05 oz.	41.28 grams

Now let's contrast this with some other foods:

Broccoli, raw, 1 cup chopped	6.04 grams
Pecan, raw, 1 oz.	4.00 grams
Beef, ground, 75% lean meat, 25% fat, patty, cooked, broiled, 4 oz.	0.00 grams
Egg, whole, raw, fresh, 1 large	.036 grams

As you can see from the examples above, some foods have lots of carbohydrates and some have few. To stay within the Lutz recommended 72 g of carbohydrates per day, some planning would be needed as there are carbohydrates in many foods. High carbohydrate foods such as soda pop would be very difficult to work into this diet.

In looking at the Lutz Diet, it has some similarities to the Specific Carbohydrate Diet. The latter diet bans many carbohydrates, which in most would most likely result in a diet with a significantly reduced carbohydrate intake level.

When I went on the Specific Carbohydrate Diet, my low iron level as measured by blood tests spontaneously increased. Dr. Lutz reported that people adopting his diet with the 72-gram carbohydrate limit experienced the same phenomena.[33] This is pretty remarkable. I'd never heard of this being a predictable outcome of any diet, but I have experienced it.

The doctors had given me prescription iron supplements from time-to-time during my sick years, and at times it was suggested that I might need iron infusions. Never ever did I hear of an opportunity to raise the iron level to normal by eating differently.

In earlier chapters, I presented some graphs that indicate the immune system level changing based on foods eaten. I suggested that eating the Specific Carbohydrate Diet will lead to the immune system operating at a higher level. Dr. Lutz appears to agree in terms of his diet. Here is what he says:

"People who eat a diet low in carbohydrates have a much stronger immune system compared to before they reduced their carbohydrate intake"[34]

This is huge. I had many conditions clear up through a diet change and believe that I now have an immune system operating at a higher level. It looks like that is what Dr. Lutz experienced with his patients. I was really surprised when I read in his book that his diet would help with diabetes.

A while back, a friend named Henry shared a story about his diabetes. Henry is in his late 70's and was experiencing difficulties controlling his sugar levels. Henry's doctor wanted him to lose some weight and stabilize his sugar at a good level.

He described the diet recommended by his doctor as a no carbohydrate diet. He eliminated potatoes, breads, fruits, and basically all foods that have significant carbohydrate content. Remaining in the diet were many vegetables and meats.

Henry did achieve the desired results. He lost some weight and his sugar level stabilized at a good level. He said his doctor called him a "non-diabetic diabetic". Henry did not have a name for the diet he was on, but it was consistent with Dr. Lutz's claim in his book as follows:

"The good news is that diabetes can be reversed by the reduction of carbohydrates in the diet."[35]

Henry is certainly a very good example of this.

Several months later, another friend of mine who lives across the country told me a similar story. Harvey was experiencing diabetes and a number of health issues, including being overweight. His doctor suggested that he significantly reduce his intake of carbohydrates. He followed his doctor's advice and to his surprise, his sugar level came into control. At the time I talked to him, he was still checking his sugar four times per day, but he no longer needed insulin. He was pretty amazed.

I recently ran into Matt, a person I've known for over 20 years. He has a history of being a little overweight, high cholesterol, high blood pressure, and diabetic. He's on a bunch of medications. He told me a story as we chatted about the turnaround in his health. With light pressure from his wife, he started to make some diet changes. With his wife's encouragement and support, Matt started to reduce his carbohydrate intake and gradually realized some results.

He had lost 10 pounds a little at a time, his high blood pressure reduced, and his high cholesterol also reduced. He then started to talk about the diabetes. His sugar had returned to normal levels. His doctor, seeing the improvements, lowered his medications. Additionally, Matt told me that his energy level was up (Matt is a retiree) and he was sleeping much better at night than he had in the last 20 years. I felt so happy for him.

Dr. Lutz in his book mentions the famous Atkins Diet. He said that his and the Atkins Diet are in principal the same.[36] Most of what I'd heard about the Atkins Diet is associated with weight loss. Maintaining a good body weight is very helpful in minimizing health issues and improving longevity. It might benefit you to take a look at the Atkins Diet and consider health effects along with better understanding its relation to the Lutz Diet.

I remember from years ago hearing a lot about the popular diet program developed by Dr. Atkins. My grandmother, who was overweight, had one of his books on her bookshelf. I doubt very much that she ever tried anything in the book, *Dr. Atkins' Nutrition Breakthrough: How to Treat Your Medical Condition Without Drugs*. This was the fifth of 17 books he published between 1972 and 2003, the year he died. The cover flap on this book says that "After caring for over 17,000 patients, Dr. Robert C. Atkins has developed a nutritional system for successfully treating physical and emotional illness without the side effects or dangerous risks of drugs."

The well-known Dr. Atkins is most remembered in the area of weight loss, but he also claimed he could help with many more health issues including insomnia, anxiety, depression, alcoholism, headache, colds and viruses, cancer, arthritis, diabetes, heart rhythm, and many more. Atkins recommended diet, vitamins, and mineral supplements as part of his program. It's not as popular now as it was when Dr. Atkins was living as he is no longer here to champion it.

With the diet being primarily remembered for weight loss, in present times it is challenged. I've known people who tried the Atkins Diet and did get good results in terms of weight loss. Unfortunately, it was not a "cure" as some thought it would be. Dr. Atkins confirmed that when he wrote that his diet "brings about weight loss, which continues as long as the diet is maintained."[37] People who achieved their weight loss goal unfortunately often returned to what they were eating before and the weight would return.

My specialist has commented several times to me over the years about the Atkins Diet with its reduced carbohydrate intake. He commented that people with bowel disease would experience a favorable impact on the bowel function and associated symptoms if they adhered to the diet.

The main point of the Atkins Diet itself is to "restrict total carbohydrate intake to the point where the body's stored fat serves as fuel."[38] Either in grade or middle school, I was told this was how the body was supposed to work. Stored fat was supposed to be the source of energy in the body. This is a subject of controversy today. Some experts say we should get our energy from carbohydrates, and some believe we should get our energy from fat.

A modified version of the Atkins Diet is now used for the treatment of children that experience seizures - that version of the diet being one that is high in fat as well as low in carbohydrates.

.

Chapter 20

The Ketogenic Diet and the Body's Need for Fat

One day, a very excited Elaine Gottschall called. That is actually an understatement. For most of the call, I just listened and she did all the talking. That was pretty typical of calls with her.

She had just received a call from Jim Abrahams, the well-known movie director and writer. Abrahams, Zucker and Zucker had been involved in a number of famous movies, including *Airplane*. The phone call was totally unexpected to her.

Elaine relayed to me that Abrahams explained that his young son, Charlie, had been afflicted with seizures. Further, his son didn't respond to the drug treatments from doctors. Given his great concern for his son, Abrahams set out to find alternate treatments or what treatments had been out there before the drugs were developed. His research led him to Johns Hopkins and the Ketogenic Diet Center in Baltimore, Maryland.

Charlie was taken to Johns Hopkins and after a review of his case, was admitted to the Ketogenic Diet program. The results were dramatic. Charlie's seizures stopped. Where the drugs had failed, the diet worked.

Abrahams told Gottschall that going forward, it was his plan to set up a foundation and get information about this diet into every hospital in the United States.

What really sparked Elaine about their conversation came up next. Abrahams told her that he believed the ketogenic diet was a sub-diet of the Specific Carbohydrate Diet that Elaine had written about in her book. The telephone call with her ended shortly afterward, but Elaine was over the moon with excitement.

To further explain Mr. Abrahams point, the Specific Carbohydrate Diet *can be* but is *not necessarily* a Ketogenic Diet.

Here's why.

I was at a restaurant recently and ran into my friend, Steve. We exchanged greetings and then he started to give me an unsolicited health update. I already knew Steve had been suffering from seizures for several years and he is also overweight. He told me that his doctor had put him on a low carbohydrate, high fat diet (Ketogenic Diet).

The seizures improved and he was losing weight. I was pleased to hear that his health was improving and wished him well.

From what I've read, adults with seizures do not do as well as children when eating the low carbohydrate, high fat Ketogenic Diet. There is no question that the Ketogenic Diet is growing in popularity for weight loss.

What is Ketosis?

The Ketogenic Diet itself is low in carbohydrates and high in fat. When the fat is high enough and carbohydrates are low enough, the body goes into a state of ketosis.

Most people in our society get their energy from carbohydrates, but a person in ketosis burns energy derived from fat. Simply put, when the body is deprived of carbohydrates, it needs another source for energy. It begins to convert fat into ketones which becomes your body's new fuel source, hence, a state of ketosis.

The Ketogenic Diet as a result is not a rigidly structured list of foods okay and not okay to eat. The diet works because of the proportions of fats, proteins, and carbohydrates result in the body going into this state.

Ketosis can be confirmed by tests, but the tests are not necessary if the diet is appropriately controlled. When the diet is used in the treatment of seizures for children, often the foods are weighed to control the proportions.

The Specific Carbohydrate Diet, the Paleo Diet, the Lutz Diet, and Atkins Diet can be Ketogenic diets depending on the specific foods and proportions eaten.

It seems logical that the benefits of each of these diets could potentially be enhanced if the Ketogenic version was followed. If scientific studies are ever done, and I am not holding my breath, this verification through study would be greatly beneficial.

History of the Ketogenic Diet

It's necessary now to go back into the origins of the Ketogenic Diet. From what I can tell, there were three treatments for seizures, especially in children, prior to the development of the Ketogenic Diet. Starting in the mid 1800's, bromides which have anticonvulsant and sedative properties, were used. In the early 1900's, another drug, phenobarbital, was developed which gained some popularity and has been in use for many years. Also, early in the 1900's, Dr. Hugh W. Conklin introduced a fasting diet. The fasting period lasted for approximately three weeks during which only water is consumed. It turned out to be very effective and became a mainstream treatment. It should be noted that Dr. Conklin was treating many other ailments as well with his water diet.

Dr. John Howland, who was among Dr. Sydney Haas' circle of professional contacts, was involved in research into understanding how the fasting worked just prior to the 1920's. He was well-known in his era and I'm including him in to show the 'small world' environment of medical doctors at this level communicating their research with each other. It is likely that these two prominent doctors influenced each other's work.

A step forward occurred in the early 1920's. It was noticed that seizures would stop in children after only a couple of days of the fasting/water diet. It was thought that a diet including food might have the same result. Dr. Rollin Woodyatt found that a diet rich in fat and low in carbohydrates produced the same effect. Another doctor, Russell Wilder, closed the loop by applying a high fat low carbohydrate diet to children with seizures, and found it to be effective. It was Wilder who dubbed the diet as the Ketogenic Diet.

This diet was added to the tool box of doctors treating children with seizures and it was used extensively. For many years, the Ketogenic Diet was the premier treatment for children with seizures, but eventually gave way to newer medications. This was the case until Jim Abrahams brought the diet into the limelight again. It has since gained much more notoriety.

The diet continues to be offered to patients and is managed through the Pediatric Epilepsy Team at Johns

Hopkins. The medical giant has been involved in its use since the diet's early development in the 1920's.

In addition to Johns Hopkins, the Pediatric Clinic at Lucile Packard Children's Hospital, Stanford University Medical Center, also takes referrals for those seeking treatment for seizures using the Ketogenic Diet. This diet has been enjoying a renaissance in recent years in the treatment of seizures in children and was likely spurred by the work of Jim Abrahams and The Charlie Foundation, which was formed after his phone call with Elaine Gottschall and still operates to this day with Abrahams its director.

Fast forward to recent years, I found an article in a journal that suggests it might help people who suffer from epilepsy, aging, Alzheimer's disease, Parkinson's disease, Amyotrophic Lateral Sclerosis (ALS, also known as Lou Gehrig's Disease), cancer, stroke, Mitochondrial disorders, brain trauma, psychiatric disorders (depression), autism, and migraines.[39]

It's interesting that researchers Carl E. Stafstrom and Jong M. Rho in an article stated, "the mechanisms through which the KD works remain unclear."[40] This diet has been part of the mainstream medical treatment since the 1920's - around 100 years! Again, more research would help in understanding why it works.

In addition to the list of conditions mentioned above, the Ketogenic Diet has been found to lead to weight loss. Bookstores are loaded with Ketogenic Diet books and recipe guides geared for people interested in weight loss.

The MAD Diet (modified Atkins Diet) based on the Atkins Diet was developed in 2002 at Johns Hopkins Hospital. MAD requires that carbohydrate intake be at very low levels such as the 10 gram to 20 gram level, and the levels of protein and fat are not limited. To strictly follow the Ketogenic Diet for an epilepsy patient, the foods must be weighed to assure the proper amounts. I stress this again because it's very important in seizure patients.

It's interesting to know that the MAD Diet was developed by Johns Hopkins as an easier-to-follow Ketogenic Diet. This would result in better diet compliance by patients.

Christy Brissette wrote an online Washington Post article titled, *Can eating fat help you lose weight? Let's look at the Ketogenic Diet.* Brissette's primary focus was weight loss. She reports that the "diet has been trending for the past three years..."[41] She offers several pros and cons for the diet including the favorable comment that "...some people find it easier to have a list of foods they can eat as much as they want of."[42] This is very similar to the Gottschall comment on weight normalization. Brissette also suggested several potential health benefits, including lowering the risk of heart disease.

The cons she presents are similar to those reported for diets other than eat anything you want. She says, "It's boring" and "There goes your social life", and that digestive woes may occur due to low fiber."[43] Journalists tend to give both sides of a story and let the reader choose. In this case, the benefits may be outweighed by the negatives, she suggested.

Both the Ketogenic and modified Atkins diets reduce the carbohydrate intake and increase the fat. Those attributes are important due to the neurological effect this way of eating has on the body - a very important benefit.

As I have pointed out, many diets can be adapted so that together they become that diet and the Ketogenic Diet. It's my belief that this is what ties the Ketogenic Diet and diets presented in the preceding chapters together.

Chapter 21

Gluten Affects Everyone

The Specific Carbohydrate Diet and Paleo Diet are gluten free. The Lutz Diet allows gluten-containing products but at a reduced level. Atkins allows so few carbohydrates in its maintenance diet that any amount of gluten consumed would be minimal. Gluten is not recommended for the Ketogenic Diet. Gluten itself is a subject that is somewhat controversial as reports disagree on whether it is good or bad for a person's health. I personally have come to the belief that foods containing gluten are not good choices.

Gluten impacts people at three levels. First, there are those that have celiac disease which is an extreme reaction to gluten. Celiac disease can be confirmed through blood testing. Second, there are those who don't have celiac disease but react to gluten anyway and are said to be gluten sensitive. Gluten sensitivity is diagnosed by ruling out celiac disease and then removing gluten to see if there's a favorable impact on symptoms. Third is the category that most people fall into, which is no obvious negative symptoms associated with gluten ingestion. No negative symptoms don't necessarily mean no impact. The percent of people impacted at the first two levels mentioned is estimated by various sources to be as high as 30%.

When we eat foods that contain gluten, compounds are formed in our digestive process that find their way to impact the brain "down to our pleasure and addiction center," according to Dr. David Perlmutter, a board-certified neurologist.[44] In other words, our brains really like gluten and gluten-containing products. From a supplier's point of view, this is a very desirable characteristic for a food item. As a result, food manufacturers like to include gluten in products because of this effect that impacts virtually everyone.

When we think of gluten, we think of digestive distress and associated symptoms found in a small percentage of the population with celiac disease. We think that for the rest of us, gluten is not an issue; in fact, we think gluten-containing foods are actually good for us.

Examples of foods that contain gluten include all wheat and rye-based products, barley, brewer's yeast and many soups, pastas, cereals, sauces, gravies, salad dressings, food coloring, and beer. In other words, gluten is not easy to avoid. Most of our population is consuming this every day, and for many, in every meal.

Brain dysfunction can be caused by the gluten-containing bread that you eat, according to Dr. Perlmutter.[45] He suggests that gluten is "one of the greatest and most under-recognized health threats to humanity.[46] Some of the disorders he suggests through studies done that implicate gluten include schizophrenia, epilepsy, bipolar disorder, ADHD, and autism.[47]

Gluten and Autism

It's widely known that many people with autism are helped by removing gluten along with dairy from the diet. Unfortunately, this diet has not been proven to be effective by studies, so it's not promoted by the medical establishment. This is another example of a diet where there is substantial anecdotal evidence that it works but has yet to be proven by research to be effective.

Some years ago, I was invited to an event in Georgia that was set up by a group of mothers of autistic children. They were interested in learning more about the Specific Carbohydrate Diet from me. I found that many of the moms already had their children on the gluten-free casein-free (GFCF) diet. I heard many success stories indicating significant improvements in their children with this diet change. A few of them told me there was further improvement with changing to the Specific Carbohydrate Diet (with the dairy removed). I left the event very convinced that the diets were a big contributor to improvement for their autistic kids. These success stories are anecdotal to the medical world, not proof.

Because of our genetic makeup, each of us is a little different. We can have different outcomes from eating the same food items. One person might have no symptoms, while another could have severe digestive distress, and another may get headaches. All these and other symptoms may have the same underlying cause. This is true for gluten and gluten-containing products.

Also, we have many conditions that don't show up until years later. I've heard the story many times of people in their youth experiencing severe sunburn and later in life getting skin cancer in that location. A person could experience no outward symptoms from eating gluten, and yet gluten potentially can silently be working on the brain and helping to accelerate the process of a disorder such as Alzheimer's.

Gluten and celiac disease are words that are often used interchangeably as the association is so strong, having been established over many years. We tend to think that if we don't have celiac disease, then foods containing gluten are just fine for us to eat. That line of thinking I believe is incorrect, as I have previously mentioned. But let's talk about some topics regarding celiac disease and celiac sensitivity. There are similar and less pronounced outward symptom impacts to so-called "healthy" people.

Celiac Disease

Celiac disease is thought by the medical community to be an autoimmune disease. Eat something that contains gluten and in a person with celiac disease, the body reacts unfavorably, often with diarrhea and weight loss. That is the first warning message, an answer from the gut, that gluten should not be eaten. It's my belief that the immune system is working correctly by sending the body a message to stop eating gluten to avoid potential damage to the body. This message should clearly be listened to.

Around 1% of the population is estimated to have celiac disease. That is 3 to 4 million people in the United States. The Beyond Celiac organization tells us that "83% of Americans who have celiac disease are undiagnosed or misdiagnosed with other conditions."[48] This is a high number, but there are blood tests for diagnosis. More blood testing would lead to more being diagnosed.

Additionally, the most insidious feature of celiac disease reported by the Celiac Disease Foundation is that "Some people with celiac disease have no symptoms at all, but still test positive on the celiac disease blood test. A few others may have a negative blood test but have a positive intestinal biopsy. However, all people with celiac disease are at risk for long-term complications, whether or not they display any symptoms."[49]

Here is another example of a disease that can afflict people that can be in a form without symptoms. Pretty scary.

In Chapter 8, there was a discussion of people being exposed to sulfur dioxide gas with some showing symptoms and some symptom free. The exposure to sulfur dioxide is bad for anyone, even in the absence of symptoms. This very important concept could extend to those who consume gluten as well. There are many children and adults who have celiac disease who do not experience symptoms and who don't realize they have it. Whether or not a person exhibits symptoms, or whether or not they have celiac disease while testing positive in the intestinal biopsy, the body is being impacted with potentially serious long-term implications.

Those people have no reason to even think they have celiac disease. Only about one-third of people diagnosed with celiac disease experience diarrhea, and about half have weight loss. Twenty percent of people with celiac disease have constipation, and 10 percent are obese. In addition to digestive problems, other signs and symptoms of celiac disease include anemia, loss of bone density, itchy, blistery skin rashes, headaches and fatigue, numbness and tingling in the feet and hands, joint pain, reduced functioning of the spleen, and acid reflux and heartburn."[50]

There have been some studies that indicate for every person diagnosed with celiac disease, there are eight who didn't know they had this condition.[51] The bad news is that many people who have celiac disease may have what seems to be unrelated symptoms or even minimal to no symptoms. As a result, they go undiagnosed. They might not realize that they have a rather significant health condition. This hits home to me as before my Crohn's disease symptoms emerged, I had many conditions that didn't appear to be bowel function related.

Gluten-free Diets

The main treatment by the mainstream medical community today for celiac disease is the gluten free diet. These is no medication available to counter the impact of gluten. Gluten-free foods are becoming more and more available. The general population, in addition to people diagnosed with celiac disease, have been creating a growing market for gluten free products.

In researching gluten-containing foods such as wheat, I didn't find anything so unique that would suggest it should be required in our diet. Breads made from wheat, especially whole wheat bread, are considered good sources of fiber and vitamins. The fiber in bread can be easily replaced with fiber from other sources such as berries, avocado, coconut, lima beans, Brussels sprouts, and nuts, among many others - all good sources of dietary fiber. The vitamins and minerals in bread can be obtained from other items as well such as vegetables, poultry, and dairy items. Bread and other gluten-containing foods can be eliminated from the diet as long as care is taken to insure the body's fiber, vitamin, and mineral needs are contained in other foods.

I don't know how many times I've heard that we need to eat whole grain bread and how good it is for us - all that great fiber! I remember the story of the woman who was on the Specific Carbohydrate Diet and explained it to her doctor. He replied that he didn't think that a person could survive without bread. He was really wrong. I have been grain-free for years and am very healthy in terms of my sense of well-being and vital signs and blood tests - in spite of my health history.

I know a woman who has eaten grain-free and has been following the Specific Carbohydrate Diet for over 20 years. She is now in her 60's and enjoys remarkably good health. She has no issues associated with her bowel disease and is medication free.

If we give up gluten-bearing wheat and other grains, there are alternatives for making bread. Recipes exist for making bread based on nut flour rather than the grains such as wheat, rice and corn. The nut-based breads to some have gourmet qualities (see Appendix B). Taste and appearance are slightly different and yet they contain fiber. Unfortunately, most groceries don't offer Specific Carbohydrate Diet compliant breads, so if a person like me wants bread, it most likely will be homemade.

People with celiac disease are often told that the cause of their disease is their body's adverse reaction to gluten. Many studies that show symptom reductions in people with celiac disease are done by excluding products containing gluten. Sounds like cause and effect. However, there is more to the story. Let's go back in history.

Dr. Sydney Haas points to Dr. L. Emmett Holt, Sr., who was the head physician at New York's Babies Hospital (which became, under his direction, the leading pediatric hospital of its time), as the person who stirred interest in the early 1900's in working towards a cure for celiac disease. Holt asked Drs. Christian A. Herter, John Howland, and Haas to work directly on this cause.[52] Each subsequently made significant contributions to this effort.

Dr. Herter was a well-known physician (co-founder in 1905 of Journal of Biological Chemistry and still in publication to this day) in the early 1900's who worked on diseases of the gastrointestinal tract. In those days, children with celiac disease often suffered from stunted growth. Dr. Herter found that increasing carbohydrates to stimulate growth led to an increase of symptoms.[53]

Dr. Howland was also a well-known physician in the early 1900's. His renown was so great that the American Pediatric Society's highest honor even today is the John Howland Award. A professor of pediatrics at Johns Hopkins Medical School, Dr. Howland reported in 1921 a treatment for celiac disease of avoidance of all carbohydrates.[54] He made this report as part of his presidential inaugural address to the American Pediatric Society. This was known to be the best approach for people with celiac disease at that time.

The Banana Diet

The major breakthrough in celiac disease was the "banana diet" first reported in 1924 by Dr. Haas in the article titled "The Value of the Banana Diet in the Treatment of Celiac Disease." Dr. Haas was a pediatrician who was dealing with children suffering from what was then known as an incurable celiac disease. The Banana Diet was "a diet in which carbohydrates except those in bananas had been excluded."[55] Haas had discovered that the carbohydrate-rich banana was well tolerated by those with celiac disease. A little-known trivia fact is that Haas' work was significant in increasing the popularity of bananas in the American diet.

Haas also went on to discover that monosaccharides (simple sugars) present in fresh fruits, honey, and numerous vegetables could be eaten by people with celiac disease. Disaccharides and polysaccharides as found in lactose (in milk), grains, and other foods when reintroduced brought on symptoms.[56]

Dr. Sidney Haas' Legacy

In 1949, there was a Golden Jubilee World Tribute at the New York Academy of Medicine to Dr. Haas, who at the time was 79 years old. The book documenting this celebration remains available even today and is titled *Golden Jubilee World Tribute to Dr. Sidney V. Haas,* published by The Committee for the Golden Jubilee Tribute to Dr. Sidney V. Haas.

It was very clear that this event was celebrating the accomplishments of a world-renowned doctor. The peer recognition through attendance at the event along with the testimonials from both attendees and non-attendees from around the world were amazing. A couple of years after this event, Dr. Haas along with his son, Dr. Merrill Haas, added to his legacy by publishing a textbook on celiac disease.

The book, *Management of Celiac Disease,* detailed the studies and the resulting Specific Carbohydrate Diet that was developed to treat celiac disease. This is the diet that Elaine Gottschall wrote about in her book, carrying the legacy of Dr. Haas forward. To this day, there is little argument that the diet is effective for celiac disease.

In 1950, the year before the father and son Haas book was published, Dr. Willem-Karell Dicke presented his doctoral thesis at the University of Utrecht Holland on the gluten free diet treatment for celiac disease. In 1953, Drs. J.H. Van de Kamer, H.A. Weijers and W.K. Dicke published the journal article, *Coeliac disease. IV. An investigation into the injurious constituents of wheat in connection with their action on patients with coeliac disease.* These publications alerted the world to the gluten free diet for people with celiac disease that would be less restrictive and still have a significant impact on disease symptoms.

While Dr. Haas' Specific Carbohydrate Diet is gluten free, it is more limiting in food choices that can be eaten. The shift towards the gluten free diet from the Specific Carbohydrate Diet began in the 1950's and remains in place today. Doctors and patients preferred an easier diet to carry out treatment.

The Celiac Disease Foundation stated, "It is estimated that up to 20% of people diagnosed with celiac disease have persistent symptoms while on a gluten-free diet."[57] The most common reason given for symptoms of celiac patients is that either knowingly or unknowingly, gluten is still being eaten. Patients are encouraged to meet with a dietitian. It could also be that these people with remaining symptoms are reacting to other foods as well.

Dr. Haas reported that, "The gluten-free diet improves the condition but does not always cure."[58] This is consistent with the idea that the gluten free diet is not totally effective for everyone. Dr. Haas was suggesting that even in the absence of gluten in the diet, symptoms remained in some patients. Haas also pointed out that in adults, celiac disease is "irreversible". Here Haas and the mainstream are consistent.

Dr. Haas treated many cases of pediatric celiac disease in his New York City practice over many years. He found that 90% of children treated with the Specific Carbohydrate Diet for a period of one year would become cured of celiac disease completely and could successfully resume a normal diet including gluten.[59] This would in fact be a true cure. However, this cure was limited to children. In adults, apparently the damage was done resulting in the permanent need to remain on the diet.

In his last years of practice, Dr. Haas had patients with bowel disorders such as Crohn's disease, ulcerative colitis, and other digestive disorders try the Specific Carbohydrate Diet. The result was very positive for patients with those diseases going into remission as well. The medical community has for years developed treatments for diseases and then tested, as Haas did, those treatments for other conditions to find any potential additional applications. Haas found the Specific Carbohydrate Diet was useful far beyond celiac disease - for Crohn's disease, ulcerative colitis, diverticulitis, cystic fibrosis, and chronic diarrhea.

The gluten free diet, applied by itself as a treatment for Crohn's disease, has not been helpful in most cases. If the medical world had not gone for the gluten free diet for celiac disease, it's likely that Dr. Haas' findings of broader application of the Specific Carbohydrate Diet would have been embraced. Unfortunately for many, that's not how it went down in history. The gluten free diet offered those with celiac disease significant relief while people with other bowel-related disorders were left to medications and operations. Also, the potential for celiac cure in children seems not to have been followed up significantly with further investigation, which is puzzling.

Dr. Haas was a dedicated doctor who was trying to find a cure for a serious ailment. Diagnosis of disease was guided by symptoms and medical tests which were much more limited in his era. The concept that there are symptom free people with celiac disease came later. In the first half of the 20th century, people were thought to be in one of two states - healthy or sick. Now we know there is a state where people appear to be healthy, but really are not with a silent disease impacting their body.

Our Food Supply

Gluten-containing crops such as wheat and barley are among the leading food crops in the United States. Other high volume food crops in the United States are corn, soybeans, oats, rice, sugar, and sorghum. All of these are leading sources of food throughout the world. No food produced from these crops are part of the Specific Carbohydrate Diet or Paleo Diet.

All these crops domestically are part of a U.S. agricultural subsidy program. It's interesting to note that many fruit and vegetable crops that are widely thought to be healthy sources of food are not federally subsidized. These subsidies for crops started before the Great Depression and continue to this day.

While these crops are important food sources to many, I am living proof that they're not needed to be healthy. In fact, eating foods from these and some other plants are likely not the best for improving our longevity and health while lowering medical care expenses.

The whole world is geared to increasing productivity in food production. Corn, wheat, rice, and other grain plants have been developed to produce crops in adverse weather conditions. Here in the Midwest where I live, we've experienced drought and excess rain and still the crops roll in. The farm equipment is refined with high capacities to harvest the crops with efficiency. Couple this with the federal crop subsidies, and a relatively stable market has been developed. While stability is seemingly a good trait, grains and some other crops in my view are not the best choice for the good health and longevity of the population.

There's an old saying that "man cannot live by bread alone". Maybe it should be revised to say, "man can live without grain-based bread."

Chapter 22

Diet Sub-optimization

Most of us don't live our lives to optimize what we eat to maximize our good health and longevity. We tend to react to trouble, especially a crisis.

When people have a health condition, doctors often suggest dietary changes. We tend to think that the *anything goes* diet is fine and no special eating pattern is needed unless there's an issue. That line of thinking is really wrong.

The Center for Disease Control and Prevention lists the major risk factors for heart disease as diabetes, overweight and obesity, poor diet, physical inactivity, and excessive alcohol use. Four of the five items just mentioned are diet or diet related. Also reported is that 23.5% of all deaths in the United States annually, the highest of all causes, are due to heart disease.

As a society, we live lives often with one or more of the listed risk factors. We somehow believe that everything is okay until we have a problem. The attitude that I've heard over and over again is that the person doesn't feel they have to make a lifestyle change. Lifestyle changes will only be considered when it's a necessity and maybe not even then. In other words, we like our foods and would rather risk disaster and hope the medical community can bail us out if we get into trouble.

In my opinion, the diets that I've covered up to this point can all be heart healthy and vital for other potential health issues. They're all better than the anything goes way of eating.

I was talking to a 49-year-old man who was experiencing high blood pressure and swelling of the ankles. Not good at such a young age. He's an example of someone who was starting to be in major trouble, but it was still early enough to turn the situation around. I really wanted to help him and made some suggestions which included the diet I eat. Like many of his generation, I received an expected courtesy thank you but knew I'd not gotten through.

The way I eat or some of the other diets I've presented likely would seem overwhelming to many, including to this fellow. I still wanted to help him, so I made a change in my approach.

I told him that there is a diet that is well regarded for use with people that have heart issues. I suggested it would be a good idea for him to get ahead on this one and change the way he eats before the doctors recommend it. The National Heart, Lung, and Blood Institute says that "DASH is a flexible and balanced eating plan that helps create a heart-healthy eating style for life."[60] While I don't believe the DASH approach is as good as the Specific Carbohydrate Diet and other previously covered diets, it's much better than anything goes. In other words, it's better to go a little in the right direction than do nothing.

Three main differences exist between this diet and the Specific Carbohydrate Diet. Unlike the Specific Carbohydrate Diet, the DASH Diet allows limited sweets, lactose from low or fat-free dairy products, and grains. I believe that all three of these are not good for a person, but heart disease shortens life more than the listed items will. It's better, but not optimal.

I don't know what the result for this young man will be since I haven't seen him since our talk. He has control of his situation though. It's up to him.

The Mediterranean Diet

Another diet I could have recommended to this young man is the Mediterranean Diet. It's gotten a lot of notoriety with a lot of books available on this subject. I once asked a medical doctor, "What is the best diet available for people to eat on an everyday basis?" The quick response was the Mediterranean Diet. This is a regional way of eating that I really knew nothing about at the time and has a good reputation relating to heart disease.

There are many reports that the Mediterranean Diet leads to increased longevity and reductions in heart issues and lower cancer rates. Foods that are commonly eaten on this diet include fruits, vegetables, nuts, legumes, potatoes, whole grains, herbs, seafood, and extra olive oil. Poultry, eggs, chicken, yogurt, and cheese are eaten in moderation. Foods to avoid include anything with sugar added, processed meat and processed foods. Minimal quantities of red meat are eaten. The dietary list is much too long to detail, but this short version should be helpful for discussion purposes.

The Mediterranean Diet offers reported opportunities for lower heart incidence and cancer rates with longer life spans. It seems similar in that regard to the DASH Diet.

Unfortunately, both the DASH and Mediterranean diets are loaded with carbohydrates (grains and others) that are hard for the digestive system to process. That certainly makes them less than optimal but a better way of eating than most people do.

Chapter 23

Putting It All Together

The digestive system is the gateway into the body for nutrition. For the body to receive and process the nutrition it needs, an effective and efficient gut coupled with foods that well match the body's needs results in good health and longevity. Failing to have the bowel function working well can be expected to impact every biological process thereafter.

The mainstream medical community does not accept the idea that diet, specifically carbohydrates, can have an impact on many digestive disorders. As a result, many subsequent recommendations and decisions by the professionals seem to me to be adverse to the health and well-being of the population.

I've demonstrated that there are diet choices which potentially impact health to a much greater degree than many realize. We need to get away from the thinking that we need a diet for each disease much like we have treatments for each diagnosis. We are all human beings and people have common nutritional needs. I believe that as a society we need to shift from the "anything goes" food approach to a standard basic diet that addresses our body's long-term needs. The diets covered in this book were intended give you some insight into potential benefits.

My pursuit into this subject is in the hopes of zeroing in on basic diet guidelines people can address for many major health issues prior to their occurrence. In other words, to delay or prevent the health problem from occurring in the first place. Our diet can become a tool we use to achieve good health and longevity.

People need to start thinking about what to do to prevent cancer, heart attack, strokes, and other major health issues. Imagine going to the doctor at age 25 and asking for direction on how NOT to have a heart attack 30 years into the future. My guess is that the doctor wouldn't know how to respond.

The need for a diet approach that could be followed by healthy and sick people alike would be useful over the years to live long and healthy lives while minimizing interventions from the medical community. If this approach could be packaged and marketed into a profitable business, it has real possibilities for a big impact.

I believe that the Specific Carbohydrate Diet developed by Dr. Sydney Haas is at the top of my list of diets for good health, followed closely by the Paleo, Lutz, and Atkins diets which have similar characteristics. These diets offer tremendous opportunities for health improvement, notably in digestive-related issues. But as discussed in this book, the impact goes far beyond digestive distresses.

To work towards establishing the effectiveness of diets, studies are needed. It's much easier to study a new medication than detailed diet plans. It's difficult for researchers to assure that diets are being totally conformed to during the periods of study, so it's not an easy task.

These diets offer potential health improvements that are not considered in the typical American diet of *anything goes*. The problem with the anything goes approach and most other mainstream diets is that they have nothing to offer for people with digestive disorders, both recognized and unrecognized.

While not generally accepted by the mainstream medical community, the ingestion of certain carbohydrates by type and quantity results in a negative impact on the body with the associated drain on the body's immune system. To confront this, the diet a person uses must address the carbohydrates.

I've read that it takes 17 years to bring a new drug to market. Numerous studies must be done and many regulations need to be complied with. If a concerted effort were started today to optimize the human diet, it would be decades before we the people would start to see the impact. That's far too long to wait, however, a trend is already underway in that direction.

Taking Charge of Your Health

In the marketplace, people subscribe to weight loss programs that are marketed by many companies. This is in reaction to having an overweight or obese condition. People buy gluten free food not only because they have celiac disease, but also as some people believe, being gluten free is a good idea.

There's a market for organic foods that purportedly contain fewer chemicals and pesticides. People will pay a premium under the right conditions. A lot of fragmentation in the "healthy food and diet" market exists so the markets to this point have remained small but growing.

The growth of the healthy food markets is an expression of the dissatisfaction with total reliance on the healthcare system. If all people were totally happy with healthcare and their resulting health, they would eat and drink anything. They could always fall back on doctors and hospitals to bail them out in tough situations.

I personally spent years in pursuit of an approach to Crohn's disease that actually works. I ended up with good health and no prescription medications by age 70 and my multitude of conditions were gone.

Our medical establishment has led our society in a heavily reactive mode in terms of health. We wait for an issue and then go to get help. What is important is what we do every single day and to move away from the reaction mode.

If a person has a single issue to address such as being overweight and wants to lose it, they need to make a change. All too often the focus is narrow on the weight issue and the long-term health is not in the game plan.

As a result, after the weight is lost, the weight returns because people want to go back to eating as usual, like they're cured. That mentality needs to change, which is much easier said than done.

The way I look at it, my health is my own personal responsibility. I'm in charge. I can call on resources to help me in my quest for longevity and health. However, I need to make the important decisions. I no longer blindly accept the advice of others. I do my homework.

The surgeries and medicines are great when the human body is injured and needs to be repaired. Advances of technologies will always be needed, especially for these cases. Our main plan for good health needs to take the form of each of us taking responsibility towards our own good health.

Longevity

How long can people live and be healthy? We really don't know. The United States Central Intelligence Agency (CIA) has a webpage listing 2017 life-expectancy-at-birth estimates for 224 countries. Leading the way is Monaco is with life expectancy being 89.4 years. On the low end is country #224, Chad, at 50.6 years. The United States comes in at 43rd place with a life expectancy of 80 years. A lot of potential improvement would need to happen for the United States to get to the Monaco level. If researchers worked hard, the life expectancy could rise to a level of over 90 or 100 years in my opinion.

I'm not talking about the 90 or 100 years of age result we get today, but healthy active people who function at 100 more like they're 50 to 70 years old. Sounds impossible, but not unlikely. If we got into the mode of serious continuous improvement efforts to achieve good health, then more and more people would live long, productive lives and the main cause of death would be wear out, commonly called old age. Resources currently dedicated to healthcare could transition over the years to other uses with some going to proactive products and services that advance the cause of good health.

Populations of people do not change all at once. As an example, the campaign to discourage smoking has been continuing for decades. There's been a big reduction in tobacco use over the years, yet it has been slow. Transitions can and do occur over time. Some people will not change, but those who do have the opportunity to reap great benefits.

The concept of prevention is what is done in advance to ward off problems from occurring in the future. Prevention in healthcare is what is done to keep minor issues and significant issues such as heart disease, cancer, and stroke from ever happening, or happening much later in life.

The foods I eat are consistent with maximizing the level of my immune system while extending my lifespan. It also minimizes minor or significant health issues. I'm no longer interested in short term food pleasures as it turns out the food I eat now, I enjoy more. The benefits of the changes I've made and propose for others may seem to border on science fiction, but it's very real and very doable.

Diets, or stated another way, "what we eat all the time" should be considered for good health and longevity. Historically, diets around the world are part of a local or regional culture based on the climate, soils, and growing seasons in the regions. Local and regional diets are often handed down from generation to generation. Many are based on the crops and livestock that thrive in those regions. Commercial businesses try to be profitable based on taste, convenience, cost, and other factors.

What we're looking for in terms of good health for people is the result. The studies and the data should all be done to get to successes which help people.

Testing According to Experts

Here I am, one of many who has successfully used the Specific Carbohydrate Diet to achieve good health. There are many of us scattered about the country. However, we're merely just anecdotes or testimonials. We're not considered to be data that is significant.

The experts always look for "proof". They like the double-blind studies where neither the observer nor the subject knows whether they're using a placebo or the proposed test. Diets are not conducive to that sort of testing regime. The studies experts want will never be done – at least not in that way, which puts the proof of the value of the Specific Carbohydrate Diet or any other diet in limbo.

Among sick people with bowel-related diseases is where the use of the Specific Carbohydrate Diet has increased in use over the years. It's really a trend. Not yet at a high level, but at a level where the media occasionally publishes or reports on this subject. It's a trend fueled by medications and operations that have given us less than satisfactory results, and in some cases, significant side effects.

The Paleo and Ketogenic diets are also part of growing trends. They're filling a void left by shortcomings elsewhere. People who have a need or have a dissatisfaction will turn to something different. It's like a fisherman throwing out the line hoping to snag a fish. The growing numbers of people trying different eating patterns have needs and wants to fulfill in their pursuit of good health.

It's time for people to start taking action to achieve good health. It's time for people to get out of the mode of reacting to health issues after they occur when the damage is already done.

While we have impressive technologies in medicines and operations, it's always better for them not to be needed. We want to have the technology around in case there are unexpected issues, but this shouldn't be the main plan.

The big debate in healthcare shouldn't be cost and how to pay for it. It should be how best to pursue good health. We as a society should be emphasizing avoiding heart disease, cancer, strokes, and other major diseases.

We should be proactive in approaching health through good lifestyle choices, including good diet.

Epilogue

I had planned on this book to include content up to my 70th birthday. So, everything that precedes this epilogue is based on that premise and it's all to the best of my knowledge true and accurate. Shortly after my 70th birthday, as I was wrapping up the book, I went in for a routine doctor appointment.

Just prior to this annual check-up, blood was drawn for the tests my physician had prescribed the previous year. It was a pretty extensive battery of blood tests. Unfortunately, this time there was a problem in one area.

My doctor looked at the results with me in disbelief. He said, "These results cannot be correct." The first step was to have the blood redrawn and get new testing, he said. Again, the results came out the same. I have a significant problem. The issue is in my kidneys; specifically, I now suffer from kidney failure. Until the diagnosis was confirmed, I had no idea of such a significant issue.

Subsequently, I've been through an extensive battery of medical testing. My heart is good, my arteries are clear, and except for my kidneys, I'm in excellent condition. The big question is, what caused the kidney failure? The doctors were unable to identify a probable root cause leaving my paperwork with "cause unknown".

Causes of kidney disease are often diabetes, high blood pressure, reduced blood flow to kidneys, illicit drugs, and prescription drugs along with several others. I had been medication free for many years so that potential cause seemed unlikely.

My primary care physician strongly recommended that I undergo a kidney biopsy to see if the root cause could be determined. I agreed at the time - it seemed like a good idea. If I were ever to have a kidney transplant, it would be good to know the cause of the kidneys failing as the same problem could conceivably damage a transplanted kidney. I approached my nephrologist (kidney specialist).

I shared with him the recommendation for the kidney biopsy. In fact, I brought it up to him three times. Each time he responded that it would be a waste of time as all that would be found is tissue from a diseased kidney. As a result, the kidney biopsy did not happen.

It was late in October when the kidney problem was identified and I was already in stage 4 kidney disease. Dialysis is required when a person deteriorates to stage 5. I had no idea that I had such a serious problem.

My condition gradually deteriorated and by early January, I was hospitalized with severe dehydration. They gave me intravenous fluids for four days and I went through a battery of blood testing prescribed by my primary care physician. Nothing significant was found and I was released from the hospital with the understanding that I would have another blood draw three days after release from the hospital.

The blood was drawn on Thursday morning and by that afternoon I had a call from the nephrologist's office telling me an appointment had been set up for me the following day. I later found out that the nephrologist normally did not have office appointments on Fridays.

The news was not good. I was advised that I needed to get on dialysis as soon as possible as I was in stage 5 kidney disease. The following Monday, I scheduled to have a permcath (hemodialysis catheter) installed and was to start dialysis on Tuesday. The nephrologist gave me his contact information in case I was unable to get through the weekend.

I made it through the weekend and the permcath was installed in my jugular vein just below my shoulder blade. The following day I received my first dialysis treatment with the machine connected to my newly installed permcath.

After a training period at the dialysis center, the first few months we tried home hemodialysis. but that proved stressful for both my wife and me. The machine has a system of alarms that trigger pretty easily. Clearing the alarms in a timely fashion was not always easy and there were fears on our part that something bad could happen to me. We gave it a good try but eventually switched to a traditional dialysis center where I had three 4-hour treatments a week.

While on dialysis, we started the process to get on the kidney transplant list. At the introductory class, we found that there is typically a four-year wait in my area for a diseased donor kidney. We filled out the paperwork to trigger the process to go forward.

I went through what seemed to be a very thorough battery of testing. These tests were to see if I was in good enough health to go through transplant surgery with a high probability of a successful outcome. I passed all the tests and no significant issues of any kind beside the kidneys were found. Following the testing, my wife and I were interviewed by various members of the transplant team. Following these processes, the transplant team met and agreed that I should be approved and put on the waiting list. Now, it looked like the wait was going to be around four years unless the perfect diseased donor match came through.

That is not the course that was followed.

Two of our daughters came forward both offering to be kidney donors for me. Both went through the blood testing and both were equal matches for me. Between them, they decided which would go forward.

Our youngest daughter went through a process similar to the one I'd gone through including physical testing and interview processes. She was approved by the transplant team. I was scheduled for a transplant in early August in the same year I started dialysis.

Live donor kidneys tend to be more successful and last longer for the recipient. We were shown charts in a class arranged by the transplant team that donors' long-term health prospects are somewhat better than the nondonor population. We figured that donors must be more health conscious after donating a kidney.

Parents spend their lives raising children and doing for them throughout their lives. I would never ask a child to be a kidney donor, but our daughters were adamant they wanted to do this. Given their high level of desire to go forward with the surgery, I agreed.

The surgery took place in August and was fairly uneventful. Both my daughter and I came through it just fine.

Initially, my blood test numbers for my new kidney were excellent. I was in the hospital for five days and then released. The follow-up schedule was pretty intense. I had blood tests and doctor appointments twice per week. Shortly after release from the hospital, the critical blood test number for the kidney started to go up. The doctor's reaction was swift. He upped my water intake, made medication changes, and had me undergo some tests. Nothing was initially found and then I went through a biopsy procedure on the newly transplanted kidney. Something was found. It was oxalate crystals on the kidney. Oxalate is the material that often make up kidney stones.

I was diagnosed with secondary hyperoxaluria. The doctor asked me if I had bowel surgery that resulted in a shortened bowel. My answer was yes. I later found out that the word "secondary" in the term secondary hyperoxaluria meant that the disorder was the result of a primary cause such as a shortened gut. A shortened gut is found in Crohn's disease patients like me and in bariatric patients who have undergone bowel shortening surgeries.

Now we had arrived at the root cause of my kidneys failing. My secondary hyperoxaluria had damaged my kidneys leading to dialysis treatments and the same issue was starting to work on my newly installed kidney.

My primary physician had been proven right about needing a kidney biopsy at the time the kidney disease was identified. The nephrologist was wrong for discounting my need for one. Secondary hyperoxaluria is somewhat rare, but I was a prime candidate. Not only was my gut shortened by surgeries, but I previously had two episodes of kidney stones. A shortened bowel does not process oxalates found in common foods as well as it would be in the length of gut we are born with. Also a factor is oxalate content in foods eaten which is the source of oxalates.

In my case, the doctors could not identify any reason why my kidneys failed, which is why the doctors should have looked further. The concern that I had was the transplanted kidney could suffer the same fate as the natural kidneys that had already failed.

Once the root cause was discovered, the post-transplant doctor prescribed a low oxalate diet and a calcium supplement before each meal. The calcium's intent is to help rid oxalates from the body. The transplant team gave us diet information from the University of Pittsburgh Medical Center (UPMC) and we immediately adopted the low oxalate diet in addition to the Specific Carbohydrate Diet. The kidney blood test number subsequently began dropping and the crisis was past. My new kidney is doing well and there are no signs of rejection.

In looking at oxalate content of foods, nuts are very high in oxalates. I no longer snack on nuts or bake with almond flour to protect my transplanted kidney. I no longer eat broccoli, green beans, strawberries, pineapple, and numerous other items. I do eat cauliflower, eggs, peas, avocado, all meats, and other items.

Elaine Gottschall always said that when people eat according to the Specific Carbohydrate Diet, a variety of foods should be eaten and excessive quantities of any one food should not be consumed. She always suggested that if the almond flour muffins are eaten, there should be a limit of 4 per day.

People with bowel disease, especially those with shortened gut and those using the Specific Carbohydrate Diet, should work with their doctors and be periodically monitored for kidney function. Before my transplant, I should have been screened for secondary hyperoxaluria. The common test is a 24-hour urine collection and a lab analysis can provide an oxalate level. A normal reading for oxalate with the 24-hour test is 25 mg/day with readings above 45 mg/day being a concern for secondary hyperoxaluria.

Had I been screened prior to the transplant and the secondary hyperoxaluria found, the transplant team would have put me on the low oxalate diet prior to surgery.

To summarize, my bowel disease, which I had proven to myself is controllable by food choices, which initially was treated with medications and operations, led to my shortened bowel. My shortened bowel coupled with eating nuts and other seemingly healthy high oxalate foods led to my kidney failure which led to a kidney transplant. I continue to have no other health issues such as heart disease, cancer, stroke, or other disorder.

As I look back on this, it only reinforces my belief that we should be starting the diet improvement efforts in children so that good health is maintained and prescription drugs aren't needed or are minimized. High blood pressure, diabetes, and many other conditions are, in my view, much less likely to ever happen if we make better food choices.

I decided to bring this book forward due to my belief that what I'm telling readers has only been strengthened by these recent experiences.

We really do need to put effort into avoiding medications and operations. With a properly directed effort, this can happen. The end result will be better health and longevity. I remain convinced that there are important answers to health and longevity that come right through the gut.

APPENDIX A

SPECIFIC CARBOHYDRATE DIET GUIDELINES

The allowed and not allowed food lists contain many well-known foods and are not intended to be a comprehensive list. Refer to Elaine Gottschall's book *Breaking the Vicious Cycle* for more details.

Allowed foods *do not* have added sugar.

Vegetables on the allowed food list should be fresh or frozen with no added ingredients.

Fruits on the allowed food list should be fresh, raw, or cooked, frozen. Canned fruit which states "canned in own juice" is acceptable with no added ingredients.

Milk (and other milk products such as half and half) is allowed as an ingredient for making homemade yogurt.

Brick cheeses found on the allowed food list are acceptable. There are additional cheeses that are allowed on an occasional basis.

As a general statement, consumption of alcoholic beverages should be minimized.

A partial list of allowed and not allowed foods begins on the next page.

Examples of allowed foods

Almonds
Anchovies
Apple cider
Artichoke (French)
Asparagus
Baking soda
Banana (ripe)
Beans (dried white navy)
Beef (fresh, frozen)
Beets
Berries of all kinds
Bourbon, occasionally
Brazil nuts
Broccoli
Brussels sprouts
Butter
Cabbage
Carrots
Cashews – unroasted
Cauliflower
Celery
Cheddar cheese
Cherries
Chestnuts
Coconut (unsweetened)
Coffee (weak black, perked or dripped)
Colby cheese
Cucumbers
Dates (loose California)
Dry curd cottage cheese
Eggplant

Eggs
Fish (canned in oil or water)
Fish (including shellfish)
Garlic
Gin, occasionally
Grape Juice
Grapefruit
Grapefruit juice
Grapes
Hazelnuts (aka Filberts)
Honey
Kale
Ketchup (homemade)
Kiwi
Kumquats
Lamb (fresh, frozen)
Lemons
Lentils
Lettuce (all kinds)
Lima beans
Limes
Melons
Mangos
Mushrooms
Nectarines
Onions
Orange juice
Oranges
Papayas
Parsley
Peaches
Peanut butter - (without additives)

Peanuts (in the shell)
Pears
Peas
Peas (split)
Pecans
Peppers
Pineapple juice
Pineapples
Pistachios
Pork (fresh, frozen)
Poultry (fresh, frozen)
Prunes
Pumpkin
Pumpkin seeds
Raisins
Rhubarb
Rye, occasionally
Scotch, occasionally
Sesame seeds
Smoothies (homemade)

Spearmint
Spinach
Squash (summer & winter)
String beans
Sunflower seeds
Swiss cheese
Tangerines
Tea (peppermint)
Tea (spearmint)
Tea (black, weak)
Tomato juice
Tomatoes
Vegetable juices (homemade)
Vodka, occasionally
Walnuts
Watercress
Wine (very dry)
Yogurt (homemade)

SPECIFIC CARBOHYDRATE DIET GUIDELINES
Examples of foods not allowed (partial list)

Foods that have a list of ingredients are likely not allowed.

Preservatives added to foods are not allowed.

Agar-Agar
Arrowroot starch
Baking powder
Barley
Bean & lentil flour
Beer
Bologna
Bouillon cubes
Brandy
Buttermilk
Carob
Carrageenan
Cheese, processed
Chocolate
Coffee, instant
Cordials
Corn
Corn bread
Corn starch
Corn syrup
Cottage cheese
Dextrose
FOS
High fructose corn syrup
Hot dogs
Ice cream
Ketchup
Liqueurs
Maple syrup
Margarine
Meats (processed)

Milk
Molasses
Oats
Pasta
Pectin
Postum
Potatoes, all types
Rice
Rum
Rye
Soup bases, instant
Sour cream
Soy bean milk
Soybean oil
Sugar (cane, beet)
Tapioca starch
Tea, instant
Turnips
Wheat
Wheat flour
Wheat bread
Yogurt (commercial)

APPENDIX B

Selected Recipes

Almond Flour Bread

The following makes a 4" x 8" loaf of bread.

Ingredients:

3 1/2 cups blanched almond flour
1/4 cup melted butter (real butter)
1 teaspoon baking soda
1/4 teaspoon salt
3 eggs
1 cup homemade yogurt fermented for 24 to 34 hours or 1 cup Farmer's cheese

Recipe steps:

Heat oven to 350 degrees F.

Completely butter the inside a 4" x 8" bread pan. Dust the inside pan surfaces with almond flour.

Mix the ingredients in a food processor or with a hand mixer.

Place the mixture in the bread pan evenly.

Bake for about 45 minutes at 375 degrees F or until a toothpick inserted into the bread comes out clean.

After the bread is baked and removed from the oven, take a knife around the edges to the bottom of the bread pan to loosen the sides of the bread from the pan.

Turn the bread pan upside down on a cooling rack and the bread will fall onto the rack, then turn the loaf of bread right side up.

Cool until room temperature and then slice. Freeze the bread that will not be eaten within a few days.

Blueberry Muffins

The following makes about 2 1/2 dozen blueberry muffins:

Ingredients:

5 cups blanched almond flour
1/2 cup melted butter (real butter)
1/3 cup honey
1 teaspoon baking soda
1/2 tablespoon cinnamon
1/4 teaspoon salt
7 eggs
1 1/2 to 2 cups of frozen blueberries

Recipe steps:

Preheat oven to 375 degrees F.

Put muffin papers in the muffin pan.

Mix all ingredients except the almond flour and the blueberries in a blender until thoroughly mixed then transfer to a bowl.

Hand mix the frozen blueberries with the other ingredients in the bowl.

Hand mix the almond flour with the other ingredients in the bowl until the mix is uniform.

Fill each muffin paper about half full.

Bake for about 15 to 20 minutes at 375 degrees F or until a toothpick inserted into a muffin comes out clean.

Cool until room temperature.

Freeze muffins that will not be eaten within a few days.

Zucchini Muffins

The following makes about 2 1/2 dozen zucchini muffins:

Ingredients:

5 cups blanched almond flour
1/2 cup melted butter (real butter)
1/3 cup honey
1 teaspoon baking soda
1/2 tablespoon cinnamon
1/4 teaspoon salt
7 eggs
2 zucchini (grated)

Recipe steps:

Preheat oven to 375 degrees F.

Put muffin papers in the muffin pan.

Mix all ingredients except the almond flour and the zucchini in a blender until thoroughly mixed then transfer to a bowl.

Hand mix the grated zucchini with the other ingredients in the bowl.

Hand mix the almond flour with the other ingredients in the bowl until the mix is uniform.

Fill each muffin paper about half full

Bake for about 15 to 20 minutes at 375 degrees F or until a toothpick inserted into a muffin comes out clean.

Cool until room temperature. Freeze muffins that will not be eaten within a few days.

Raisin Muffins

The following makes about 2 1/2 dozen raisin muffins:

Ingredients:

5 cups blanched almond flour
1/2 cup melted butter (real butter)
1/3 cup honey
1 teaspoon baking soda
1/2 tablespoon cinnamon
1/4 teaspoon salt
7 eggs
1 package of raisins

Recipe steps:

Preheat oven to 375 degrees F.

Put muffin papers in the muffin pan.

Mix all ingredients except the almond flour and the raisins in a blender until thoroughly mixed then transfer to a bowl.

Hand mix the raisins with the other ingredients in the bowl.

Hand mix the almond flour with the other ingredients in the bowl until the mix is uniform.

Fill each muffin paper about half full.

Bake for about 15 to 20 minutes at 375 degrees F or until a toothpick inserted into a muffin comes out clean.

Cool until room temperature.

Freeze muffins that will not be eaten within a few days.

Vanilla Yogurt Ice Cream

The following makes a little over 4½ cups of ice cream:

Ingredients:

1/2 cup honey
1 1/2 teaspoons vanilla
1/8 teaspoon salt
4 cups homemade yogurt fermented for 24 to 34 hours - it is recommended to make the yogurt using half and half to help enhance the taste

Recipe steps:

Mix the ingredients with a hand mixer.

Follow the directions on your ice cream machine.

Freeze the ice cream that is not immediately eaten.

Cauliflower "Potato" Salad

The following makes 4 to 6 servings:

Ingredients:
1 large head of Cauliflower
4 hard-boiled eggs, peeled and chopped
1 cup finely chopped celery
½ cup finely chopped onion
1/3 cup chopped dill pickle
¼ cup homemade mayonnaise
¼ homemade yogurt (fermented for 24- 34 hours)
2 teaspoons of apple cider vinegar
2 teaspoons of plain mustard
1 teaspoons of salt

Recipe steps:

Chop cauliflower and steam until tender. Drain well. When cauliflower is cool, chop into bite sized pieces.

Mix together with the homemade mayonnaise and homemade yogurt.

Mix in vinegar, plain mustard and salt.

In a large bowl, mix this with the cauliflower pieces. Add the celery, onion, and pickle. Mix the egg in last.

Chill in the refrigerator. Flavors taste best after being chilled for several hours or more.

Mayonnaise

Ingredients:

2 egg yolks
2 tablespoons apple cider vinegar or fresh lemon juice
2 tablespoons water
1 teaspoon honey
1 teaspoon dry mustard

¼ teaspoon salt
1 cup olive oil

Recipe steps:

Place egg yolks in a container and mix with a hand blender.

Add the vinegar, water, and olive oil and mix thoroughly.

Add the honey, salt, and mustard and mix thoroughly.

Store in the refrigerator when not in use.

Homemade Yogurt Instructions

The following makes 2 quarts.

Ingredients:

2 quarts whole milk, or 2% milk, or 1% milk, or half and half or other similar product (avoid ultra-pasteurized and added ingredients).

Yogurt starter (1/2 cup of good quality commercial yogurt or powdered yogurt starter per the manufacturer's instructions)

Recipe steps:

If water is used by the yogurt maker, put in warm water and turn the unit on.

Pour the milk product into a pan.

Heat the milk product to 180 degrees or bring to a simmer while stirring constantly. The lower the fat content of the milk, the more likely it will scorch on the pan.

Remove the milk product from the heat a couple of minutes after temperature has been achieved.

Cool the milk product until 110 degrees is achieved. An ice water bath can be used.

After the temperature has gone down to 110 degrees, thoroughly mix with the milk, the powdered yogurt starter or commercial yogurt.

Pour the mixture into the yogurt container and put on the cover.

Put the yogurt container(s) into the yogurt maker and cover for the 24 to 34-hour fermentation cycle.

Once the fermentation is complete, put the yogurt into the refrigerator for 4 to 8 hours to allow it to set up. The yogurt will keep for up to 3 weeks in the refrigerator

Additional Reading

Anible, Kathryn. *Baking for the Specific Carbohydrate Diet: 100 Grain-Free, Sugar-Free, Gluten-Free Recipes.* Ulysses Press, 2015.

Bager, Jodi. aging *Grain-Free Gourmet.* Whitecap Books Ltd., 2010.

Bager, Jody and Lass, Jenny. *Everyday Grain Free Gourmet: Breakfast, Lunch & Dinner.* Whitecap Books Ltd., 2010.

Conrad, Kendall. *Eat Well, Feel Well: More Than 150 Delicious Specific Carbohydrate Diet™-Compliant Recipes.* Clarkson Potter, 2010.

Gottschall, Elaine. *Breaking the Vicious Cycle: Intestinal Health Through Diet.* Kirkton, Ontario: Kirkton Press, 1994.

Haas, Sidney V. and Haas, Merrill P. *Management of Celiac Disease.* Philadelphia: J.B. Lippincott Company, 1951.

Hagood, Natalie and Roberts, Jenna. *Cooking to Heal Little Tummies.* SCDiet.com, 2008.

Kerwien, Erica. *Cooking for the Specific Carbohydrate Diet: Over 100 Easy, Healthy, and Delicious Recipes that are Sugar-Free, Gluten-Free, and Grain-Free.* Ulysses Press, 2013.

Lipp, Sherry. *Don't Skip Dessert: Gluten-Free, Grain-Free & Sugar-Free Sweet Treats.* Lulu.com, 2013.

Prasad, Ramon. *Adventures in the Family Kitchen: Original Recipes Based on the Specific Carbohydrate Diet.* SCD Recipe LLC, 2004.

Prasad, Ramon. *Colitis & Me: A Story of Recovery.* SCD Recipe LLC, 2003.

Prasad, Raman. *Recipes for the Specific Carbohydrate Diet: The Grain-Free, Lactose-Free, Sugar-Free Solution to IBD, Celiac Disease, Autism, Cystic Fibrosis, and Other Health*

Conditions. (Healthy Living Cookbooks). Fairwinds Press, 2008.

Prasad, Raman. *The SCD for Autism and ADHD: A Reference and Dairy-Free Cookbook for the Specific Carbohydrate Diet.* Swallowtail Press, 2015.

Ramacher, Sandra. *Healing Foods - Cooking for Celiacs, Colitis, Crohn's and IBS.* Amazon Digital Services LLC, 2015.

Rosset, Lucy. *Lucy's Specific Carbohydrate Diet Cookbook.* Lucy's Kitchen Shop, Inc., 2010.

Spencer, Beth. *Turtle Soup: Recipes for The Specific Carbohydrate Diet from An SCD Mom.* Muskegon, Michigan: Beth Spencer Fine Arts, 2011.

Sweeney, Tucker and Thompson, Carol. *Two Steps Forward, One Step Back: A Journey.*

Through Life, Ulcerative Colitis, and the Specific Carbohydrate Diet. CreateSpace Independent Publishing Platform, 2011.

Weiss, Rochel. *A Taste of Wellness.* 2013.

About the Author

Over his lifetime, John E. Chalmers experienced numerous chronic health challenges. Faced with these issues, through research and extra effort, he found ways to overcome seemingly insurmountable obstacles through food choices.

Chalmers and his wife, Cheryl, reside in Indiana where he spends much of his time in retirement and is involved in his community.

Endnotes

1. U.S. Department of Health & Human Services, National Institutes of Health, https://www.nih.gov/about-nih/what-we-do/budget (accessed August 2, 2017).

2. Margot Sanger-Katz, "When Hospitals Buy Doctors' Offices, and Patient Fees Soar" New York Times, February 6, 2015.

3. https://www.nytimes.com/2015/02/07/upshot/medicare-proposal-would-even-out-doctors-pay.html (accessed August 2, 2017).

4. Margot Sanger-Katz, "When Hospitals Buy Doctors' Offices, and Patient Fees Soar" New York Times, February 6, 2015.

5. Gerald Imber, M.D., Genius on the Edge: The Bizarre Double Life of Dr. William Stewart Halsted (New York, February 2011), 6-7.

6. Amy Schlaes, Coolidge, (Toronto, ON, February 2013), 327.

7. Strobes, Mike. "No clear cause of drop in US life expectancy", Fort Wayne Journal Gazette, December 9, 2016, section A, 9.

8. Strobes, Mike. "No clear cause of drop in US life expectancy", Fort Wayne Journal Gazette, December 9, 2016, section A).

9. Gary E. Fraser, Diet, Life Expectancy, and Chronic Disease Studies of Seventh-day Adventists and Other Vegetarians (Oxford University Press, New York, 2003) 58.

10. Gary E. Fraser, Diet, Life Expectancy, and Chronic Disease Studies of Seventh-day Adventists and Other Vegetarians, 58.

11. Gary E. Fraser, Diet, Life Expectancy, and Chronic Disease Studies of Seventh-day Adventists and Other Vegetarians, 58.

12. Laura J. Stevens, Complete Book of Allergy Control (Pocket, March 1986), 11-13.

13. Laura J. Stevens, Complete Book of Allergy Control, 129.

14. John Trowbridge, M.D., and Morton Walker, D.P.M., The Yeast Syndrome (New York, Random House, May. 2011), 4.

15. Natalie Golos and Frances Golos Golbitz, If This Is Tuesday, It Must Be Chicken, or How to Rotate Your Food for Better Health (Keats Publishing, July 1983).

16. Radon and Cancer, American Cancer Society, https://www.cancer.org/cancer/cancer-causes/radiation-exposure/radon.html (accessed August 2, 2017).

17. Elaine Gottschall, Food and the Gut Reaction (Kirkton Press, March 1992).

18. Drs. Sydney V. Haas and Merrill P. Haas, Management of Celiac Disease (J.P. Lippincott Company, Philadelphia, 1951).

19. Elaine Gottschall, Breaking the Vicious Cycle: Intestinal Health Through Diet (Kirkton Press, July 1994), 27.

20. Elaine Gottschall, Breaking the Vicious Cycle: Intestinal Health Through Diet, 29.   National Institute of Diabetes and Digestive and Kidney Diseases, Overweight and Obesity Statistics, https://www.niddk.nih.gov/health-information/health-statistics/overweight-obesity (accessed August 17, 2017).

21. National Institute of Diabetes and Digestive and Kidney Diseases, Overweight and Obesity Statistics.

22. About CCFA, Crohn's and Colitis Foundation of America. http://online.ccfa.org/site/PageNavigator/tof15_about_ccfa.ht ml (accessed August 15, 2017).

23. Crohn's and Colitis Foundation of America, Diet and Nutrition.

24. Journal of Gastroenterology and Nutrition, THE SPECIFIC CARBOHYDRATE DIET - A TREATMENT FOR CROHN'S DISEASE? Fridge, J. L.1; Kerner, J.1; Cox, K.1. June 2004 - Volume 39 - Issue - pp S299-S300, http://journals.lww.com/jpgn/Fulltext/2004/06001/P0637_th e_Specific_Carbohydrate_Diet___A_Treatment.761.aspx (accessed August 15, 2017).

25. Journal of Gastroenterology and Nutrition, P0637 THE SPECIFIC CARBOHYDRATE DIET - A TREATMENT FOR CROHN'S DISEASE? Fridge, J. L.1; Kerner, J.1; Cox, K.1. June 2004 - Volume 39 - Issue - pp S299-S300.

26. Journal of Pediatric Gastroenterology and Nutrition, January 2014;58(1):87-91, titled Nutritional therapy in pediatric Crohn disease: the specific carbohydrate diet by D.L. Suskind, G. Wahbeh, G, N. Gregory, H. Vendettuoli, and D. Christie. https://www.ncbi.nlm.nih.gov/pubmed/24048168 (accessed August 16, 2017).

27. Loren Cordain, PhD., The Paleo Diet Revised Edition Lose Weight and Get Healthy by Eating the Foods You Were Designed to Eat (Houghton Mifflin Harcourt (2011), 71-74.

28. Loren Cordain, PhD., The Paleo Diet Revised Edition, 91.

29. Loren Cordain, PhD., The Paleo Diet Revised Edition, 99.

30. Christian B. Allan, Ph.D. and Wolfgang Lutz, M.D., Life Without Bread: How a Low-Carbohydrate Diet Can Save your Life (McGraw-Hill, July 1, 2000), 5.

31. Christian B. Allan, Ph.D. and Wolfgang Lutz, M.D., Life Without Bread, 7.

32. "USDA Food Composition Databases", United States Department of Agriculture, Agriculture Research Service, https://ndb.nal.usda.gov/ndb/search/list (accessed September 4, 2017).

33. Christian B. Allan, Ph.D. and Wolfgang Lutz, M.D., Life Without Bread, 120-121.

34. Christian B. Allan, Ph.D. and Wolfgang Lutz, M.D., Life Without Bread, 209.

35. Christian B. Allan, Ph.D. and Wolfgang Lutz, M.D., Life Without Bread, 34.

36. Christian B. Allan, Ph.D. and Wolfgang Lutz, M.D., Life Without Bread, 203.

37. Robert C Atkins, M.D., Dr. Atkins' Nutrition Breakthrough: How to Treat Your Medical Condition Without Drugs, New York, Perigord Press (1981) 271.

38. Robert C Atkins, M.D., Dr. Atkins' Nutrition Breakthrough: How to Treat Your Medical Condition Without Drugs, 271.

39. Carl E. Stafstrom and Jong M. Rho, "The Ketogenic Diet as a Treatment Paradigm for Diverse Neurological Disorders". Front Pharmacol. 3:59.

40. Carl E. Stafstrom and Jong M. Rho, "The Ketogenic Diet as a Treatment Paradigm for Diverse Neurological Disorders".

41. Christy Brissette, "Can eating fat help you lose weight? Let's look at the ketogenic diet", Washington Post, September 26, 2016.
https://www.washingtonpost.com/lifestyle/wellness/can-eating-fat-help-you-lose-weight-lets-look-at-the-ketogenic-

diet/2016/09/23/096ab83a-7f50-11e6-8d13-
d7c704ef9fd9_story.html?utm_term=.0cc524284b65
(accessed August 17, 2017).

42. Christy Brissette, "Can eating fat help you lose weight?
Let's look at the ketogenic diet", Washington Post, September
26, 2016.

43. Christy Brissette, "Can eating fat help you lose weight? Let's
look at the ketogenic diet", Washington Post, September 26,
2016.

44. David Perlmutter, M.D., Grain Brain (Little, Brown and
Company, New York, Sept. (2013) 64.

45. David Perlmutter, M.D., Grain Brain, 4.

46. David Perlmutter, M.D., Grain Brain, 32.

47. David Perlmutter, M.D., Grain Brain, 32.

48. Beyond Celiac, Celiac Disease Fast-Facts,
https://www.beyondceliac.org/celiac-disease/facts-and-
figures/ (accessed August 17, 2017).

49. Celiac Disease Foundation, Celiac Disease Symptoms,
https://celiac.org/celiac-disease/understanding-celiac-disease-
2/celiacdiseasesymptoms/ (accessed August 17, 2017).

50. Donna M. Weir, Strange Body Common Autoimmune
Disease Questions Answered, (lulu.com, May 24, 2014), 200.

51. Thalheimer, Judith C., RD, LDN, "Silent Disease", Today's
Dietician, May 2014, p22.

52. Sidney V. Haas, M.D., "Celiac Disease", New York State
Journal of Medicine, May 1, 1963, Vol. 63, No. 9: 1346.

53. Haas, "Celiac Disease", 1346.

54. Haas, "Celiac Disease", 1346.

55. Sidney V. Haas, M.D. "Celiac Disease", New York State Journal of Medicine, May 1, 1963: 1347.

56. Haas, "Celiac Disease", 1347.

57. Celiac Disease Foundation, Celiac Disease Follow Up and Treatment, https://celiac.org/celiac-disease/understanding-celiac-disease-2/treating-celiac-disease/ (accessed August 17, 2017).

58. Sidney V. Haas, M.D., "Celiac Disease", New York State Journal of Medicine, May 1, 1963, Vol. 63, No. 9: 1350.

59. Sidney V. Haas, M.D., "Celiac Disease", 1349.

60. "Description of the DASH Eating Plan", U.S. Department of Health and Human Services, National Heart, Lung, and Blood Institute, https://www.nhlbi.nih.gov/health/health-topics/topics/dash (accessed August 20, 2017).

Index

5
5-day rotation diet, 43-45, 48

A
Abrahams, Jim, 129, 132
ADHD, 136
aging, 85, 132
airborne allergies, 37, 46, 60, 61, 62, 63, 64, 100, 113
Allan, Christian, 140
allergies, 40, 43, 44, 58, 100, 110
Alzheimer's disease, 132
American Cancer Society, 57
American Pediatric Society, 140
Amyotrophic Lateral Sclerosis, 132
anemia, 80, 124, 138
ankylosing spondylitis (AS), 28, 77, 100
antibiotics, 10, 12, 73, 77, 78, 111
arthritis, 128
AS. See Ankylosing Spondylitis
asthma, 23, 110, 113
Atkins, 110, 130, 133, 134, 135, 136, 139, 150
Atkins, Robert C., 135
autism, 120, 132, 136
autoimmune diseases, 36, 59, 79, 106, 137

B
banana diet, 140
biofeedback machines, 26
blood pressure, 110, 127
Body Mass Index, 70
bowel disease, 48, 64-65
Breaking the Vicious Cycle, 62, 89, 90, 173
bronchial asthmatic, 23
bronchitis, 110, 11

C
cancer, 5, 17, 53, 78, 80, 84, 85, 87, 105, 114, 124, 128, 132, 137,146, 147, 152, 159
CCF. See Crohn's Colitis Foundation (CCF)
celiac disease, 62, 106, 124, 135, 138, 140-142, 150
Celiac Disease Foundation, 137, 142
Center for Disease Control and Prevention, 145
Central Intelligence Agency, 152
Charlie Foundation, 132
cholesterol, 110
colitis, 36, 40, 77, 80, 93, 99, 106, 142
Conklin, Hugh W., 131
constipation, 138
Cordain, Loren, 119, 120
Crohn's Colitis Foundation (CCF), 93
Crohn's disease, 30, 33, 37, 38, 40, 47, 56, 58, 62, 67, 77, 79-83, 86, 89, 91, 94, 98, 100, 106, 120, 138, 142, 143, 151, 158

D
Daniel Plan, 117, 118
DASH, 146, 147
depression, 127, 132
diabetes, 84, 114, 123, 126-128, 145, 155, 160
Dicke, Willem-Karell, 141
disaccharide, 63
Dr. Lutz, 124

E
enteritis, 38
epilepsy, 131, 132, 136

F
failure costs, 15, 16, 17
food allergy, 37

185

Made in the USA
Las Vegas, NV
22 December 2020

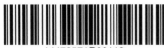

14473571R00118